"As a pediatrician, I now see more cases of 'almost autism' than I do autism itself. These neurodevelopmental challenges continue to rise at an alarming rate, and parents need answers. Maria provides those solutions in the most thorough yet conc... uide to healing the body and the ... on natural and nutritional solu... and her specific recommendatio... ory therapies provide parents w... the roadmap they need ... eat Sensory Processing Disorder.

— Bob Sears, MD, FAAP, author of *The Autism Book* and *The Allergy Book*

"*Almost Autism* is a much-needed bridge between the biomedical and sensory aspects of spectrum disorders. It is important reading not only for parents, but also for occupational and speech therapists, educators and anyone guiding families toward health."

— Patricia Lemer, author of *Outsmarting Autism: The Ultimate Guide to Management, Healing and Prevention*, Chairman of the Board, Epidemic Answers

"*Almost Autism* is a compelling personal story that is also a comprehensive guide to recovering your child from Sensory Processing Disorder. Hong's narrative is accessible, easy to read, and a practical resource for parents who are overwhelmed and confused by their child's behaviors and symptoms. If you are a parent of a child affected by SPD, or any of the 'new childhood epidemics,' this book should be your companion and guide while on the road to recovery."

— Beth Lambert, Executive Director of Epidemic Answers, Executive Producer of the Canary Kids Project and author of *A Compromised Generation: The Epidemic of Chronic Illness in America's Children*

"Maria has thoughtfully provided a comprehensive map that will guide you through the haze of medical misinformation surrounding an SPD diagnosis. With her practical step-by-step guide, you will leave the fog behind and step into a higher place of clarity and health; not just for your kids, but your whole family! Get started, today!"

— Lisa Joyce Goes, co-founder of The Thinking Moms' Revolution, President, teamTMR.org

"In *Almost Autism*, Maria Rickert Hong has given us a book of amazing depth and scope that explores the complex and often-misunderstood condition knows as 'Sensory Processing Disorder.' What makes this book stand out is the way in which she carefully deconstructs the causes of SPD and offers a systematic biomedical approach to treatment, offering options without overwhelming parents. Clearly this comes from her personal connection to this problem as well as her extensive professional expertise. As a holistic developmental pediatrician, I will be recommending *Almost Autism* as an invaluable resource to many of my families."

— Stephen Cowan MD, FAAP, author *Fire Child Water Child, How Understanding the Five Types of ADHD Can Help You Improve Your Child's Self Esteem and Attention*

"Maria explains Sensory Processing Disorder and its many facets – the signs, causes, underlying pathophysiology, and treatments - in a way that is easy to understand, well organized and practical to both the layman and health care provider. Maria's guidance has been essential in helping me recover my own child's health as well as mine; and I will most certainly be using her book as a reference for my medical practice!"

— Melissa Crawford, MD, CCFP

"Maria Rickert Hong has managed to write a clear, understandable, yet comprehensive roadmap for parents struggling to help their children. In her fight to heal her own sons she left no stone unturned, and readers not only benefit from reading about her experience, but also are given tools to help in their own struggle. *Almost Autism* is a tale of hope and a manual for healing."

— Vicki Kobliner, MS, RDN, co-author of *A Compromised Generation: The Epidemic of Chronic Illness in America's Children*

"*Almost Autism* will benefit any parent whose child suffers from complex or overlooked health conditions. Maria Rickert Hong shares tremendous insight, science, and practical advice stemming from her personal experience and professional study. She provides detailed methods for making sense of multi-faceted symptoms and the broad array of therapeutic approaches. From defining the condition, to understanding the causes, to navigating helpful solutions, this book covers it all. I highly recommend *Almost Autism* to families struggling with Sensory Processing Disorder, autism, and other developmental delays."

— Julie Matthews, BS, NC, author, *Nourishing Hope for Autism*

"Finally someone has put together in one book everything I've been trying to tell parents about, but don't have time for in a homeopathy consultation, plus so much more. On every single page I wanted to jump up and down and shout 'Every parent has to read this book!'"

— Begabati Burke Lennihan, RN, CCH, author of *Your Natural Medicine Cabinet: A Practical Guide to Drug-Free Remedies for Common Ailments*

"Finally Sensory Processing Disorder is explained in a way that takes into account its complexity AND the multiple intertwined factors involved in overcoming it. Parents who are 'in the trenches' working to recover their children from SPD and related disorders will benefit enormously from this in-depth, yet highly readable book."

— Sonia Story, Neurodevelopmental Movement Educator and Owner, MovePlayThrive.com

"If you have a son or daughter with autism, Sensory Processing Disorder or ADHD/ADD, this is a must-read book. It will open your mind to new possibilities on how to help these children. By Maria's own fierce determination and passion to help her sons, she now offers countless tools to change the lives of these precious children."

— Ellen W. Cutler, DC, founder of ECM, author of *Clearing the Way to Health and Wellness*

"Forthright and clear, Maria begins with a warning to parents: environmental toxins including vaccines do contribute to neuro-developmental disorders, allergies and more in children. After recovering her own children from Sensory Processing Disorder, Maria put to paper the practical steps she took, outlining the dietary interventions and therapies that helped or worked. If you are faced with a similar diagnosis of SPD in your child, this is the book for you."

— Heather Fraser, author of *The Peanut Allergy Epidemic: What's Causing It and How to Stop It*

"The book *Almost Autism* illustrates how complicated what I call autism and Maria refers to as a Sensory Processing Disorder can be. Maybe we should just stop calling it autism because what we are seeing is not really autism at all but a medical condition where each child must have their individual medical issues addressed in order for recovery to happen. Although each of us wants the one cure fits all or that magic bullet, it just doesn't exist. Trust me, I searched everywhere for it. The solution is never easy and recovery results from many things. For my son, recovery involved medical, behavioral and educational interventions combined. As parents we hate how long recovery takes. But it does happen. Maria's story demonstrates that kids do get better and gives families hope for their children's future. Parents must NEVER GIVE UP until they find the right answers for their children!"

— Marcia Hinds, Ryan's mom and author of *I Know You're In There, Winning Our War Against Autism*

"Maria Rickert Hong has written a detective story, a passionate account of her journey in helping her boys get their health back from 'almost autism,' or Sensory Processing Disorder. She has also written a well referenced, eminently useful and comprehensive guide on how we can all stay healthy in the 21st century-suitable for parents and practitioners alike."

— Marvin Schweitzer, ND, founder of The Wellness Institute, Norwalk, CT

"Maria Rickert Hong has delivered an incredibly insightful book on the crisis occurring in our children. Her book, *Almost Autism*, is a must read for parents struggling with an atypically developing child. She tackles difficult and controversial topics in a manner that makes sense and empowers parents to take action in guiding, supporting and fixing their children's development in every area, from what they eat to how they move and how they look. Her references are exhaustive and readers will be impressed with her knowledge and understanding of the challenges parents face."

— Randy L. Schulman, MS, OD, FCOVD, co-author of *Envisioning a Bright Future: Interventions That Work for Children and Adults with Autism Spectrum Disorder*

"This is the definitive go-to manual for what to do if you are concerned that your child is behind in meeting any developmental milestones. Maria provides a comprehensive summary of the most effective interventions available and while these approaches ARE backed by science, they are not commonly discussed in the media. Your own doctor may not even know about them.

This is the book that I needed 8 years ago when my child was diagnosed with auditory and visual processing disorders and a mild form of dyslexia. Thankfully the holistic approach we also adopted worked to completely recover my child - but this book would have saved me hours of time and angst."

— Pauline O'Sullivan, mother of three, Director Victus Health Trading Pty Ltd., Australia

"*Almost Autism* is not just a book, but an actual tool that parents and caregivers can use to help their children recover from Sensory Processing Disorder and other chronic illness. Ms. Hong presents thorough research to back up the myriad root causes of illness including environmental factors as triggers for neurodevelopmental disorders followed by a comprehensive description of solutions. A must read for parents of children with chronic illness and anyone that wants their child to have the healthiest, best start in life."

— Michelle Giliberto, co-founder of Epidemic Answers, Reiki master, energy healer and vibrational therapy practitioner

"*Simply loved it!* In many years as a holistic health practitioner and as a mother, I applaud this book! Full of wisdom, knowledge and facts. A realistic view of a problem facing our nation and many families. A must read and gift to your doctor."

— Ma Prem Jothi Samadhi Sandra, soul doctor

Almost Autism:

Recovering Children from Sensory Processing Disorder, A Reference for Parents and Practitioners

MARIA RICKERT HONG, CHHC, AADP

Westport, CT

www.MariaRickertHong.com

Printed in the United States of America.

Library of Congress Control Number: 2014917922

ISBN: 978-0-9909041-0-6

DEDICATION

To my sons who are my teachers,
and to all of our Canaries in the coal mine,
thank you for taking on this burden
and showing us that we need to be healed.

DISCLAIMER:

This content is not intended to be a substitute for professional medical advice, diagnosis, or treatment. Always seek the advice of your physician or other qualified health provider with any questions you may have regarding a medical condition. Information provided is for informational purposes only and is not meant to substitute for the advice provided by your own physician or other medical professional. You should not use the information or products contained herein for diagnosing or treating a health problem or disease, or prescribing any medication. Information and statements regarding alternative health products have not been evaluated by the Food and Drug Administration (FDA) and are not intended to diagnose, treat, cure, or prevent any disease.

CONTENTS

ACKNOWLEDGMENTS

Kathleen DiChiara, thank you for being my cheerleader.

Joshua Rosenthal and Lindsey Smith of the Institute for Integrative Nutrition, thank you for helping me turn this idea into a reality.

Patricia Lemer, thank you for being my mentor and taking me under your wing.

Beth Lambert, thank you for allowing me to put my passion to work and spread the word that recovery is possible.

INTRODUCTION

I've written this book for you because I don't want you to go through the same struggle I did. I have recovered both of my sons from Sensory Processing Disorder, what I call "almost autism.". I believe Beth Lambert, the Executive Director of the Epidemic Answers non-profit and the Canary Kids Project where I work, may have coined the term. It refers to the fact that there are so many overlaps and similarities between autism and Sensory Processing Disorder (SPD). In fact, SPD is one of the hallmarks of autism, but a child with SPD isn't necessarily autistic.

When my boys were younger, I struggled to understand why this was happening. I didn't get much help from pediatricians, and I think a lot of that has to do with the fact that SPD is not a diagnosis – yet. But I think it also has a lot to do with the fact that most pediatricians aren't aware of common underlying causes of SPD, autism, ADHD and other neurodevelopmental disorders. These causes are toxicity, gut dysbiosis, immune dysregulation, nutritional deficiencies, hormonal imbalances and inflammation, among others, and I'll go into more detail about them later in the book.

Recovering Your Child from "Almost Autism"

If doctors don't understand the causes, how can they possibly help your child? That's where I come in with this book. I'm going to show you that by doing what's called a "biomedical approach," which means addressing these causes, as well as specialized therapies, it's possible that your child can also recover from SPD. I'm not guaranteeing it, but I think you should at least give it a shot.

It took me years of working with my naturopath, Dr. Marvin Schweitzer, working with specialized therapists and doing my own research into these causes for me to understand how all of this fits together. I'll show you how the puzzle pieces come together in this book and help you unravel them as well. There is no silver bullet for the cause of "almost autism," and there's no silver bullet for recovery, either. Each person has been affected differently by their exposure to foods, toxins and other stressors.

My biggest "aha" moment came when I read Dr. Kenneth Bock's book, *Healing the New Childhood Epidemics: Autism, ADHD, Asthma, and Allergies: The Groundbreaking Program for the 4-A Disorders.* Although he didn't specifically mention SPD, I began to understand it by looking at the root causes, although I've added a few more in here that he doesn't mention. In any case, it was exciting to know that children can recover from autism, ADHD, asthma and allergies. If they can recover from these, then why not SPD? In fact, my children not only recovered from SPD, but also from developmental delays, hypotonia, acid reflux, eczema, failure to thrive and asthma. We're still working on mitochondrial dysfunction, hypothyroidism and adrenal fatigue, which I'll show you are also underlying factors in SPD, but at least I know how to manage these issues now.

That's what I want you do, too. Even though much of the research I point you to in this book may be specifically for autism or ADHD, I want you to understand that the causes I've mentioned underlie all of these conditions. So, if a research article mentions autism or ADHD, I want you to think that it's likely the case for children with Sensory Processing Disorder, as well.

How I Got Into This

For those of you who don't know me, I am a Certified Holistic Health Counselor trained at the Institute for Integrative Nutrition as well as the Media Director for Epidemic Answers and our Canary Kids Project. My goal is to teach people how to become advocates for their own and their children's health by educating them to think for themselves and continue to ask questions. I always tell my clients that I'm going to take their world and turn it upside down. After reading this book, you probably won't look at the world in the same way. In fact, you may find that it's hard to convince your family and friends of this, and that's typical. People don't want to change, and by you taking the steps to recover your child, you will have to change, and your friends and family may not like that and may not be supportive. That's very common and very typical. But you know what? That's OK because there's a whole new world out there of people like us who get it, and there's a growing number of us, too. You may feel like you're going through this alone, but I promise you that you aren't.

I got into this because I was forced into it by my sons' problems. Before that, I was an equity research analyst on Wall Street covering the gaming, lodging and leisure sector and the oil services sector at Salomon Smith Barney, Lehman Brothers, Jefferies & Co. and Calyon Securities (Credit Lyonnais) in New York City. And before that, I got my MBA from Tulane University while working as a marketing specialist for Halliburton Energy Services in New Orleans. How different my life is now!

Listening to Your Intuition

I would not have achieved this level of success in recovering my sons' health if I had listened to what my western, allopathic doctors were telling me carte blanche. I urge you to question what they tell you and to research health issues for yourself. I also urge you to listen to your intuition. I urge you to listen to that small, still voice inside of you. If it weren't for parents, especially mothers, listening to their intuition, where would the human race be today?

I knew there was something wrong with my sons, but I just couldn't put my finger on it. Again and again, different doctors told me, "He's fine" and "There's nothing to worry about." They said this even when I told them that my older son would throw up after almost every meal and even though his weight percentile was declining. They told me that because his height percentile was growing – for a few months – that there was nothing to worry about. They were wrong.

I would say, "My son barely eats; he eats two spoonfuls of yogurt and five Cheerios, and it takes him an hour to eat, and then he throws it all back up." They would say, "He's fine, don't worry about it." They said that all the way from his beginning at the 40th percentile for weight until he fell all the way down to the 3rd percentile at 18 months, when he lost weight. THEN they said, "There's a problem." Really!?!

I would say, "He has poor motor skills. His first crawling happened when he was eight months old, and he slithered backwards. Then, he army-crawled until he was 19 months old. He cross-crawled for only a couple of weeks before he began to walk at 20 months." All along, they were saying, "He's fine; don't worry about it." Until he hit 18 months, THEN all of a sudden they said, "There's a problem."

I would say, "He projectile vomits, and my clothes, his clothes, his car seat, chairs and rugs are covered with it constantly. He throws up after every meal." They said, "He's got a weak gag reflex; he'll grow out of it." They said this until he was 2 ½ years old, and THEN they said, "He has acid reflux. Give him some Prevacid®."

I would say, "He's hypersensitive to sounds, lights and motions. He cries all the time. Something is wrong." They would say, "He's fine; he'll grow out of it." By this point, my son was three years old, and I had had enough of being told that, "He's fine. There's nothing to worry about. He'll grow out of it."

The truth is, there was a gnawing feeling inside of me that "something's not right, something's not right." I couldn't put my finger on it. So, even though my then pediatrician du jour said, "Don't worry about it; he'll grow out of it," I had grown a pair by then and learned to put my foot down for my child.

I badgered her with questions until finally she gave up and said that maybe we should see a developmental psychiatrist. We did, and voila, we got the diagnosis (even though it's not an official DSM – the *Diagnostic and Statistical Manual* of psychiatric and mental illnesses – diagnosis) that my son had Sensory Processing Disorder.

From then on, nothing could stop us. I began to research WHY he was like this. Therapy obviously helped, but there was more to it. Why was he sick all the time? Why had he had so many ear infections? Why did he develop asthma? Why did he have developmental delays and acid reflux? Why was he so sensitive? Nobody that I knew really knew, so I had to keep digging and digging until I got to the point where I figured it out. It's toxicity, gut dysbiosis, immune dysregulation, nutritional deficiencies, inflammation and hormonal imbalances.

Unless you're one of the lucky few with an integrative pediatrician, you'll never hear that answer, despite a multitude of peer-reviewed medical research journal studies out there that they just don't have the time to read.

The system is broken. If you want health and recovery for yourself and/or your children, you will need to take your health back into your own hands and stop giving away your power. In my own experience, I have found that there is no one practitioner, not even me, with all the answers.

You need to listen to your gut instinct when it tells you that something is wrong.

It's so easy to push that knowing down and stuff it aside and listen to the authorities who tell you that nothing is wrong and don't worry about it. I'm telling you don't do it; you'll regret it if you do.

I teach my clients to become their own and their children's own advocates. If you don't do it, who will? You can't expect that someone else will care more about you and your children than you do.

My children and I would not have recovered from our health problems if I had not listened to my intuition, that little voice that said, "Something's wrong."

It's been very hard going through this, as most people, even most doctors, don't know about the causes of all these problems. Most of them don't understand that all of these problems are related, and most of them certainly don't know that recovery is possible.

We got a lot of help from changing our diets and seeing a naturopath, a functional-medicine doctor and a holistic nutritionist, as well as from me doing never-ending research about how all of these problems are connected and from special therapies I'll tell you about later.

We've recovered from so much, although there is still more work to be done. In any case, we are so much better off now than we were a few years ago, when all of these problems hit a crescendo, and I fell off the cliff with my own health problems, as many special-needs moms do.

I want people to know that recovery is possible, which is why I joined Epidemic Answers and later the Canary Kids Project. We seek to educate parents about the causes of these problems as well as let them know that recovery is possible from autism, SPD, ADHD, allergies, asthma, autoimmune and more.

In fact, we're making a documentary film to show the world that recovery is possible because most people just don't know that. Most people don't know that a child can recover from autism or asthma or that an adult can recover from an autoimmune disease, even multiple sclerosis or rheumatoid arthritis. If you want to learn more about our film project, you can visit our website at www.CanaryKidsMovie.com. If you want to find out more what it takes to recover, you can visit the Epidemic Answers website at www.EpidemicAnswers.org and my site at www.MariaRickertHong.com.

Our kids are the canaries in the coal mine, and they are showing us how toxic our world is. By understanding what is happening with them, we can heal ourselves as well. They are our teachers, and for this I am grateful.

DISCOVERING THE PROBLEM

If I were to tell you that both of my sons used to have Sensory Processing Disorder (SPD), you might: a) ask, what is that? b) ask, how did you know that they had it? or c) not believe me unless you had met them, especially my older son, a few years ago. I believe that they are recovered because of naturopathic medicine, dietary changes and occupational therapy interventions. My goal here is to help other parents understand what SPD is and what can be done about it.

It's hard for parents to put a finger on what's going on with their child – it was for me. To everyone else, your child may seem fine, but to you, because you're with him or her all the time, you notice that something is a little off. Talking to your pediatrician about it isn't likely to help as there is no official diagnosis for Sensory Processing Disorder in the *DSM-V: The Diagnostic and Statistical Manual of Mental Disorders.*

Sensory Processing Disorder can be a standalone, unofficial diagnosis, but it is also common in children with autism, pervasive developmental delays and ADD/ADHD. In addition, children can often be misdiagnosed with ADD/ADHD instead of SPD because it's not as well known.

Learning About Sensory Processing Disorder

Children with SPD have a problem with the wiring from their nervous system to their brain; Sensory Processing Disorder is a neurological disorder. SPD is usually more noticeable in kids; most adults have learned to compensate.

There are two kinds of children with SPD: sensory seekers and sensory avoiders. Sensory seekers are the kids that are constantly seeking stimulation. They like to crash hard into things or people, or they won't stop spinning or swinging. In addition, some people can be a combination of sensory avoiders and sensory seekers.

My sons were both sensory avoiders, so I can tell you more about that because of my personal experience. The most mundane things can over-stimulate sensory avoiders. Lights are too bright, sounds are too loud, the lightest touch can hurt, food textures can bother them, and motions can make them dizzy or sick. Many autistic children also have SPD.

Sounds Too Loud

A parent may start noticing that something is a little off with their SPD child because he or she cries and gets upsets at loud noises when other children aren't bothered by it. It's one of the first indications of sensory dysfunction.

Loud or unexpected noises would make my older son cry when he was a baby. It was so bad that I had to remove the batteries from any toy that made noises because he would always cry when the toys made sounds. A client of mine, a young boy, couldn't even go outside because the sound of bugs flying was deafening to him.

Lights Too Bright

Many children with SPD become upset or irritated when lights are too bright. Fluorescent lights are particularly annoying to them because of their harsh glare and humming noises.

I couldn't take my older son grocery shopping because the bright fluorescent lights, eye-catching colors, different smells, and loud, echoey noises would get to him, and he would start crying. If I was lucky and had my husband with me, he could take him out to the car to calm down while I finished shopping. If I didn't, we'd have to suffer through.

Motions Over/Understimulating

For a sensory avoider, motion avoidance and motion sickness are common byproducts of a dysfunctional vestibular sense, which is controlled by the tiny cilia inside the ears. Children who are sensory seekers LOVE the stimulation of motion. They're the kids that are constantly spinning and crashing into things.

My older son would always cry when going for a ride in the car when he was a baby. Looking back now, I'm sure it was motion sickness; he would vomit a lot when going for a ride. Even as a baby, he would cry if I put him in a swing. He refused to go on slides or merry-go-rounds. This became a real concern for me when he started preschool. I realized that if he were always to play in the sandbox while other kids played on the playground, he would never be able to make friends, and a lifetime of social isolation seemed to be a real possibility.

Food Texture Preferences

A lot of kids with SPD prefer certain food textures over others. Some like crunchy foods because it gives them the sensory input that they're looking for, while others prefer mushy foods because they lack the ability to chew properly. In fact, these children may have an oral-motor problem that prevents them from moving, chewing and swallowing properly. Some of these children may have a tongue tie and may also have problems with lisps and other speech impediments.

Sensitivity to Smells and Tastes

Because of nutritional deficiencies, especially zinc, as well as neurodevelopmental damage, many SPD kids have a profound dislike for many tastes and smells, even if they don't seem strong to anyone else. This sensitivity can lead to a downward spiral of picky eating that further exacerbates nutritional deficiencies. These days, in my experience, it's the norm that most kids, not even just those with SPD, are picky eaters; you'll find them living on cheese pizza, yogurt, chicken nuggets, Goldfish crackers and French fries.

Touches Over/Understimulating

Sadly, some SPD kids can't stand to be touched, hugged or cuddled. Bathing and washing up, even if gently done, can be difficult because these actually hurt some kids. Tags and socks with seams can bother these kids, too. My older son would cry every time I would bathe him because the sensations were just too much for him. On the flip side, other SPD kids need the extra reinforcement of touch, and you'll find them crashing into people for the extra sensory input.

Over/Undersensitivity to Pain

SPD kids can have varying tolerances to pain. Some of them cry endlessly at the tiniest little bump or scratch, while others seem to barely notice it, if at all. When my older son was younger, he had an ear infection for a while, but I never noticed it because he didn't complain at all that his ears hurt. I've had ear infections before, and I know they are excruciatingly painful.

Delay in Potty Training

Children with SPD often have difficulty understanding

their body's inner signals because they have faulty wiring of their interoceptive sense, which is their awareness of their body's functions, including those of the bowel and bladder. Many of them are four or five years old, if not older, by the time they are fully potty trained.

Apraxia/Dyspraxia

Apraxia is the total loss of motor planning, whether it's gross motor or speech, and many SPD kids have either or both of these disorders. Dyspraxia is a partial loss of motor planning. SPD kids know what they want to do or say, but because of neurodevelopmental damage, have trouble actually doing that. For example, a child with apraxia of speech may have trouble saying sounds, syllables, and words because the brain has problems planning to move the lips, jaw and tongue that are needed for speech.

Anxiety

It's not a coincidence that kids with Sensory Processing Disorder have a lot of anxiety; this is probably one of the more interesting and unknown aspects of neurodevelopmental disorders. It's stressful having a damaged neurological system. Think about what it's like when you're really trying to concentrate on something and the music or TV is too loud and the lights are too bright. It's pretty irritating, right? Imagine being like this ALL the time.

My older son had an incredible amount of anxiety. Here's an example of his anxiety for which I had horrible guilt for many Christmases: When my older son was a little over two years old, I went to my husband's Christmas party and left our caregiver to put my son to bed, something no one else had ever done before. When we got home late that night, our caregiver told me that he cried so hard over the fact that mommy wasn't there that he threw up the whole time I was gone.

Crying All the Time

Your relatives, in-laws and friends probably think you're spoiling your child because he or she cries all the time, and you'll likely feel that they're criticizing your parenting skills either behind your back or maybe even to your face. It's not your fault! These kids can't process their senses correctly, and they have a lot of anxiety because of it.

For us, it all hit the fan when our caregiver left to have her own baby shortly after my older son turned three. My older son had been used to having either me or the caregiver completely to himself. All of a sudden when she left, he was forced to share me with his baby brother. So what did he do? He cried. And cried. And cried. And cried. And cried. Over EVERY little thing.

We couldn't take him anywhere! While other kids were having fun going to birthday parties and social events, we'd try to go and then have to leave because he would cry at all the overstimulation. Even being around a lot of people would be overstimulating because of all the movement and noise.

Clinginess

A small child with anxiety clings to his or her mom or dad for calmness and reassuring. This can get taken to extremes with an SPD kid because of his or her constant anxiety about different sounds, lights, smells, motions and situations. My older son didn't walk until he was 20 months old, and before that, he was a barnacle. I felt as if he were permanently physically attached to me. It wasn't so bad when he was younger, but after his brother was born when he was 21 months old, it was extremely difficult to deal with two small, crying children at the same time, who both wanted to be picked up and held at the same time. I would feel so guilty about neglecting his little brother, and then I would get angry because it just wasn't right that the older one's needs should be taking away from the little one's. He was older, all of his peers were becoming more self-sufficient, and I didn't yet understand the impact of what he was going through.

Difficulty Transitioning

All that anxiety can lead to a child who has difficulty transitioning. It can be difficult just to go from the car to inside the house because the environment has changed. What was accounted for is now something new and potentially dangerous or upsetting. A child who has difficulty transitioning can tantrum for a loooong time, way beyond what is typical for a child of the same age.

Controlling Behavior

Because a child with SPD feels so out of control of his or her senses, he or she can become like a little dictator with routines and demands. If demands aren't met, usually by the parents, then it's hard for these children to calm down. My older son was scared to be in his own body, especially because of his vestibular dysfunction, and he became a tyrant during his bedtime routine. It was at least 20 minutes long aside from bathing, changing and brushing teeth. His routine had to be performed in a certain sequence or else he would become very upset, and I'd have to start all over again.

Refusal to Play on Playground Equipment

Refusing to swing on swings, slide on slides or go on a merry-go-round are signs that your child could have a vestibular dysfunction. The motion is too upsetting for them, kind of like when you've had too much to drink and the room is spinning. For us, it was hard to go on playground playdates because my kids wouldn't play!

Delayed Social Development

It's typical that SPD kids have difficulty relating to their peers. I'm sure that I would, too, if I had trouble processing my senses correctly! It's hard for them to judge motions and speeds of other kids, so they tend to avoid others. Both my sons played by themselves at playgroups and preschool, usually by digging holes in the dirt or sand, when they should have been engaging in parallel or associative play.

Another sign that something was off was that, although at home my older son was either a chatterbox or a non-stop crier, at preschool, he kept to himself and rarely said anything; he was incredibly withdrawn with his peers. He was so quiet his teachers thought he might have a speech problem, which he definitely didn't. Of course, once he came home, he let all of his frustration and anxiety out, as kids do, but I began to sense that the amount of his crying was far greater than that of his peers.

Having Developmental Delays

Children with Sensory Processing Disorder typically have delays in the development of gross and fine motor skills, and this is no coincidence as we dig into the causes of their neurodevelopmental damage later in this book. These delays are the typical milestones that your pediatrician is looking for such as rolling over, sitting up, crawling and walking. Later on, you may discover that your child has problems drawing or writing at an age-appropriate level.

At six months of age, my older son had problems sitting up unassisted. I used to put my nursing pillow behind him for support. Then, he didn't crawl when he should have. Instead, he slithered backwards at eight months of age. He army crawled for another eleven months, and he only cross-crawled for a few weeks.

My oldest son didn't walk until he was 20 months old and my youngest didn't until he was 16 months old. I'm not the worrying kind of person, but once both had passed the 15-month mark without walking, I really began to worry.

Our pediatrician continually reassured me that everything was "fine" and not to worry because I was just another "first-time mom who didn't know anything and worried too much." Does this sound familiar to you? I'm guessing if you're reading this, you've probably been told this by quite a few of your children's doctors.

Noticing Other Unusual Symptoms

What I always thought was odd was that not only did my sons have all these different sensory issues, but they also had a huge host of other red flags that something was wrong with their health. Pediatricians always blew off my concerns saying either that my boys would grow out of whatever the problem was or that it was no big deal. It WAS a big deal, and I encourage you to pay attention to your child's other symptoms.

In my work with Epidemic Answers and the Canary Kids Project as well as my own research beforehand, I now know that these red flags are quite common, but this is by no means an exhaustive list. Your child may have other unusual symptoms that you can't put your finger on. Following are some typical other red flags that SPD kids have.

Hypotonia

Low muscle tone, or hypotonia, can be a sign of a vestibular dysfunction as well as mitochondrial dysfunction. Mitochondria are the powerhouses of the cell, and they are often gunked up by environmental toxins. Mitochondrial dysfunction is common in children with neurodevelopmental disorders, as well as anyone with a chronic disease or disorder. I'll go over what mitochondrial dysfunction is and what you can do about it in more detail later in the book.

My older son had hypotonia to the extent that he was like a little limp rag doll. It was so sad to see other kids happily and busily playing and climbing while my son sat there like a lump on a log. In addition, both of my sons would also fall out of their chairs for no reason. Just "plop" and they would fall over onto the floor because of their low muscle tone and vestibular dysfunction.

Projectile Vomiting/Colic/Acid Reflux/GERD

A problem keeping food down is very, very common in kids with Sensory Processing Disorder. In fact, it's a risk factor for later developing SPD, autism, ADD/ADHD, OCD, ODD as well as allergies, asthma and autoimmune disorders. That's because the intestinal tract houses most of the immune system, makes most of the body's neurotransmitters, is responsible for nutrient absorption and is one of the primary routes of detoxification. When the gut is unhappy, the rest of the body is unhappy.

My sons had a long history of acid reflux problems. When my older son was a baby, he would constantly projectile vomit, and he had been projectile vomiting since he was a newborn. The doctors told me this was normal, that he was just a fussy baby with colic.

When my younger son was born, he, too, was "fussy" and "colicky." He had an outright problem with nursing: he refused to. When he would nurse, he would shriek in pain or fill up so much (probably because he was starving) that he would throw it right back up. This wasn't a little "spitting up"; this was projectile vomiting, and I had become used to having stains on the rug, chairs and clothes that simply wouldn't come out.

In the meantime, my older son continued to vomit after almost every meal and Pediasure® feeding. His throat lining was so worn out that even crying or coughing too hard, which he did a lot, would make him throw up. He was like an endless vomit machine.

When I took my older son in for his 2-1/2-year checkup, I mentioned to the pediatrician that typically when my son was sick, I wouldn't give him Periactin, which his pediatrician had prescribed to help him gain weight, as there was no sense in stimulating his appetite if all that coughing was going to make him throw up that much more. One time, however, I continued to give him Periactin, and noticed that he didn't throw up as much. I asked the doctor if that was perhaps because the medicine relaxed his throat muscles? That's when a light bulb went off in the doctor's head, and he said, "He's got acid reflux. Here, try this Prevacid®." The Prevacid® worked immediately, and my son's weight steadily improved.

When my younger son was 10 months old, it dawned on me (I'm a little slow sometimes!) that he probably had acid reflux, too. I made a list of symptoms to convince the pediatrician. My son:

- Shrieked so much when he was a newborn that the lactation consultant suggested that reflux could be a cause.
- Cried and shrieked when he was lying down to have his diapers and clothes changed.
- Projectile vomited whole bottles of milk four or five times.
- Spat up two ounces of milk about an hour after he woke up from his morning nap. He hadn't eaten anything for a few hours and was simply playing on the floor.
- Preferred smooth-textured foods.
- Frequently gagged on pastier and lumpier foods. It became worse with stage three foods.
- Refused to eat more frequently. Like feeding his brother before, it became an hour-long song and dance to get him to eat.
- Used to have a constant chest rattle/noise when breathing, even though he wasn't sick.
- Had poor weight gain as well, although not as bad as his brother's.

These are all classic symptoms of acid reflux/GERD. Guess what? The pediatrician didn't think my younger son had acid reflux. He said, "Just because his older brother has it doesn't mean he has it, too."

I made an appointment with the local pediatric

gastroenterologist, and he didn't believe it, either. Many of the moms at the playgroups were saying how their kids had acid reflux with the same symptoms, and their doctors (including the same pediatric GI) were handing out reflux meds like it was candy. Why wasn't my son getting the help he needed?

Instead, the pediatric GI wanted to do an exploratory endoscopy. Although it was an outpatient procedure, it required that my son be put under anesthesia. I felt as if I had no other choice, so I agreed. Guess what? He had acid reflux. It took all that to confirm what I already knew.

Difficulty Feeding

You can imagine that if a child has trouble keeping food down that he or she may not want to eat, as he or she likely associates pain with eating. For us, it was incredibly hard – no, "TORTURE" is the right word here – to feed my older son any solid food.

It became extremely hard for me to feed him solid foods later on when I introduced them when he was five months old. It would take a good, solid hour just to get a few Cheerios and Yo-baby yogurt in him. Then he would turn right around and throw it up. I did anything I could to distract him to get some food in him: sing, dance, have him play with toys and objects, turn on the TV or radio. None of these really worked, but I was desperate. Many times he would outright refuse to eat, but then he would be starved for his next meal. Other times he would eat some, but then he would wake up screaming and/or wake up vomiting.

It got so bad that I – being a former analyst – made a spreadsheet to show the doctor that he was only eating 10 cheerios and one ounce of yogurt a day when he was about nine months old. The rest of his calories came from breastfeeding. Any food or breastmilk I managed to get into him was typically vomited up immediately. I was told by the doctor to limit the milk to 20-24 oz. per day in hopes that this would encourage him to eat more solid food. That didn't work. He just ate less and cried even more, probably because his blood sugar was always tanked and he was starved.

I was told by the doctor that his feeding strike may be because his teeth were coming in. His teeth came in, and many times after that, he still refused to eat. I was told by the doctor to give my son gas drops, Orajel™ and Tylenol® because maybe he was gassy and maybe his teeth and gums hurt, but these didn't help.

The older he got, the longer his naps got. I suppose that because he wasn't getting enough calories to remain active, it was easier for his body to just rest when he could, although many times he couldn't rest because he would wake up cranky and/or vomiting.

My younger son had difficulty nursing because he wasn't latching on well. He would scream and shriek because he was either so hungry or because he was in pain.

Picky Eating

Children with SPD are often picky eaters for two reasons. One, they may have an oral sensitivity with a preference for certain textures, and, two, they often have a zinc deficiency which causes them to avoid foods with certain tastes or smells. In any case, picky eating begets picky eating, and a downward spiral of only eating cheese pizza, French fries and other junk food typically ensues.

Failure to Thrive

You can see how a child with acid reflux, difficulty eating and picky eating might gain weight poorly. Other reasons for failure to thrive can be mitochondrial dysfunction and subclinical cystic fibrosis, which a vibrational remedy practitioner discovered was another reason for my older son's poor growth.

I could scream every time someone tells me that I'm not that big or my husband's not that big, so my sons' failure to thrive is something I shouldn't worry about. I'm NOT comparing my boys to other kids. I'm comparing them to THEMSELVES. That's the point of a growth percentile curve. A child is born at a certain height and weight, which puts them on a growth-percentile curve, and they should track that curve. Otherwise, what's the point of having these curves?

But a mom knows when something's not right. It shouldn't take an hour to feed a child only to have him throw it all up. He ate and drank an average of 715 calories per day; he should've been getting around 1,300 on average. An average of 60% of his calories came from milk, and this didn't seem right. I was waved off – this was not the first time this was to happen – as if I were just another neurotic, hypervigilant, first-time, New York City mother.

With no help from the doctor except for a list of fattening foods to give him such as butter, cheese, full-fat yogurt and maple syrup, I desperately tried to up the calories in every bite. Dairy and sugar seemed to be the best choices for calorie loading, but I wasn't keen on giving him too much sugar. I am hypoglycemic, and I know that sugar can only exacerbate blood sugar issues by temporarily creating a short-term blood-sugar high, only to have it come crashing down quickly afterwards with the shakes, a headache, irritability and excessive body heat. So I gave him quiche, yogurt, cheese pizza, bagels and cream cheese, and any food I could think of that I was supposed to avoid for causing me to pack on pounds. Still, none of these foods helped him gain weight.

We moved to the suburbs when my older son was almost a year old. Again, the new pediatrician didn't seem concerned about his weight or vomiting. "It's a weak gag reflex; he'll grow out of it", was what I was told, despite the fact that it was continuing to take an hour to eat a meal and my son threw up almost every meal.

This went on until my son was 18 months old. That is far too old for him to have been before the doctor became concerned. By this point, my son STILL wasn't walking, he was STILL throwing up almost every meal, and his weight had dropped to the 3rd percentile from the 40th percentile and his height to the 30th percentile from the 75th percentile.

Finally, this new pediatrician was concerned. He prescribed two bottles of Pediasure® a day and said to take him to McDonald's to fatten him up on junk food. What? This was just so wrong, but I did it anyway. Do you know what? My son would barely touch the junk food, although he did pound the Pediasure®. I'll go over why this was such bad advice later in the book.

By his 2nd birthday, his weight and height bounced back to the 20th and 75th percentiles, respectively, but my son continued to throw up after every meal. It wasn't until he was 2-1/2 that the pediatrician decided that he wasn't growing out of his "weak gag reflex" and put him on Prevacid®, which worked instantly. He also prescribed periactin, an anti-histamine that has the side effect of increasing hunger; it's often given to anorexic teenage girls. In any case, the Prevacid® worked immediately, and my son's weight steadily improved.

In those days, I wasn't thinking yet. Just as the doctor ordered, I gave my kids junk food and junk drinks to help them grow and gave them pharmaceuticals to cover up their symptoms. All of that changed after I began seeing a naturopath for myself and discovered how unhealthy these things were.

My younger son, who loves to be called "Crane Man" (because he likes crane trucks), was born at the 50th percentiles for height and weight. He stayed on these curves until he was well over three years old. By the time he had been most of the way through his first year of preschool, though, his weight had declined to the 30th percentile and his height to the 41st by his 4th birthday. He was gluten-free/dairy-free for a whole year and a half before his weight percentile declined, so lack of dairy didn't seem to be the reason for his growth decline. By the time his 5th birthday rolled around, Crane Man had almost finished his 2nd year of preschool, and his weight and height had again decreased, this time to the 22nd and 14th percentiles, respectively.

Tongue Tie

It's possible that your SPD child has a tongue tie, which means that the movement of the tongue is restricted by a short, thick frenulum, the membrane that connects the tongue to the bottom of the mouth. A tongue tie can make it difficult for your child to nurse, eat or speak clearly.

Many practitioners miss tongue ties that are more subtle, called "posterior tongue ties." If you bring your child to most doctors, dentists, even lactation consultants, they may not even know what a posterior tongue tie is, let alone know how to look for it. I recommend that you check out the following websites for more information:

- Tongue Tie: www.tonguetie.net
- Lawrence A. Kotlow, DDS, PC: www.kidsteeth.com
- Loving Our Guts: www.lovingourguts.com/tongue-tie-2/

If your child has failure to thrive, a tongue tie may be one of the causes because "if the tongue is not going up to the roof of the mouth when a person swallows; the sphenoid bone does not rotate properly and growth hormones are not being released from the pituitary gland."[1]

In addition, there's a theory that tongue ties are related to a genetic defect, known as the MTHFR mutation (a methylation defect), which I'll go over later. A child with a methylation defect has trouble detoxifying, so toxins may have something to do with this epigenetic change. For more information, check out the blog post on MTHFR.net, "The Intersection of Tongue Tie & MTHFR".[2]

---

1. http://articles.mercola.com/sites/articles/archive/2013/04/07/orofacial-myofunctional-therapy.aspx. Accessed September 14, 2014.
2. http://mthfr.net/the-intersection-of-tongue-tie-mthfr/2014/05/23/. Accessed September 14, 2014.

Red Cheeks, Lips or Ears After Eating

Redness in cheeks, lips or ears after eating is a sign of a food sensitivity, intolerance or allergy, and it's a pretty common thing in SPD children. The cause is typically a sensitivity to foods containing phenols and/or salicylates, as was shown by Dr. Ben Feingold, the developer of the Feingold diet. Food sensitivities occur because of a compromised immune system, and I'll discuss the cause of that – gut dysbiosis – later in the book.

Allergic Shiners

I see so many kids running around these days with dark circles, known as allergic shiners, under their eyes; SPD kids and kids with other neurodevelopmental damage as well as those with allergies, asthma and autoimmune conditions are most likely to have them. Their cause is due to low adrenal function and backed-up lymphatic drainage.

Ear Infections

Multiple ear infections are also common in these kids, and it's not uncommon for their doctors to remove their adenoids and/or tonsils. Ear infections are a risk factor for later developing SPD, autism, ADD/ADHD, allergies, asthma and autoimmune conditions. Giving children antibiotics only compounds the reason why they're getting ear infections in the first place: gut dysbiosis. My older son had three ear infections by the time he turned two.

Chronic Constipation/Diarrhea

Because most of the immune system is in the gut, and the gut is a major route of detoxification, a child with chronic constipation/diarrhea typically has a compromised immune system and has trouble getting rid of toxins. SPD kids typically have chronic constipation/diarrhea, which are often two sides of the same coin. Often, poop gets so impacted that the only thing that can come out is water poop: diarrhea.

The problems are that most doctors wave it off as "toddler diarrhea," think that pooping a few times a week is normal (you and your child should poop at least once a day!) or prescribe dangerous laxatives like Miralax® instead of looking for the root cause of gut problems, which is gut dysbiosis. I'll discuss the dangers of these laxatives later in the book.

My older son was on Miralax® for the whole time that he was on Prevacid®, yet his pediatrician never discussed how being on Prevacid® could constipate my son and never reviewed the dangers of either one of these common drugs to my child's health.

Constant Sickness/Allergies

Most children with Sensory Processing Disorder have a compromised immune system, for reasons I just discussed. Because of this, these kids are either sick with colds all the time or have chronic allergies or sinus infections. It's all related, and it's a sign that something is wrong with your child's health if you're constantly giving him Claritin®, even if it's just for seasonal allergies.

I couldn't take my older son anywhere when he was a baby/toddler because he would get sick without fail. When he started preschool, he would be there for a week, get sick, then be out for a week because he was sick; the preschool didn't want kids coming in who were sneezing and coughing. This pattern continued constantly until I took him to our naturopath when he was four years old.

Food Allergies, Intolerances or Sensitivities

Food allergies, the kind for which your child needs an Epi-pen, are common in children with SPD, autism,

ADD/ADHD, allergies, asthma and autoimmune disorders. Think about it, though: when did this kind of allergy, like the one to peanuts, become so common that you can walk into any classroom in any school these days and know that there's a high likelihood that at least one of those children has a severe, anaphylactic allergy and needs an Epi-pen? It wasn't like that when I was a kid, and I'll be discussing the reasons for this increase in this as well as in other chronic childhood disorders when I tell you about the causes of these disorders.

In addition, there are other types of allergies, called sensitivities and intolerances, other than the kind that immediately make you break out in a rash or need an Epi-pen because you're going into anaphylactic shock. These don't cause immediately visible reactions but instead work on a subtler level to cause inflammation. Symptoms from these can take up to two to three days to appear and can vary from pain, headache, constipation, and trouble paying attention.

In our own experience, one of the pediatricians did send my older son to a pediatric allergist at Mount Sinai Hospital in New York City to look at possible food allergies when he wasn't gaining weight well, but all of the skin-prick tests came back negative. However, not one word was mentioned about sensitivities or intolerances; I didn't discover these until my older son was four and I took him to my naturopath.

Cradle Cap

Cradle cap often gets dismissed as just a nuisance that babies have, but it's a sign of a fungal infection, typically *Candida*, which means that the baby has gut dysbiosis. SPD kids often had cradle cap when they were babies. For some reason, most doctors don't think of a *Candida* infection as a diagnosis, much less a root cause of so many health problems. My older son had cradle cap when he was a baby.

Bloody or Painful Diaper Rashes

Diaper rashes seem to be blown off as just something that babies have, but if they are painful or bloody, they are warning signs that your child likely has a fungal infection such as *Candida*. My younger son constantly had painful, bloody diaper rashes. This concern was dismissed as nothing to worry about, and I was only told to put liquid Maalox® on it to lower the acidity that was literally eating at my son's sensitive skin.

Eczema

Eczema is very common in children with Sensory Processing Disorder, as well as in children with autism, PDD-NOS, ADD/ADHD, allergies, asthma and autoimmune disorders. Eczema is also a sign of a fungal infection, typically *Candida*. Western medicine treats eczema with damaging and dangerous steroids like cortisone, and I'll explain later in the book why your child should avoid them.

Asthma

It's common that a child with asthma initially started off with eczema. What most people, including Western doctors, don't realize is that suppressing eczema with cortisone or other steroids drives the disease process deeper. If the body can't use the skin as an organ of elimination, it causes the infection to go deeper into more vital organs like the lungs, and the infection becomes more dangerous as it does.

When my older son was four years old, he had a severe asthmatic episode after we went to Los Angeles to visit my husband's family. We woke up the first morning after we landed in LA to discover that the whole valley where his parents lived was engulfed in smoke from forest fires in the San Gabriel Mountains. They stayed on fire the entire week we were there, and, although we didn't go out in the smoke too much, we couldn't help but breathe in some of it in.

When we came back home, he had a severe asthmatic attack, which he had never had before. It was so bad that our new pediatrician called on a Saturday morning to see if he was OK. I didn't like having him on the nebulizer, Xopenex, albuterol and prednisolone because I knew that steroids suppress the immune system as well as cause growth delays.

Sleeping Problems

It is very common for children with SPD as well as those with other neurodevelopmental disorders to have difficulty going to sleep and/or staying asleep. Many of these children don't make enough melatonin because their serotonin production is off because they may have gut dysbiosis, poor digestion and nutritional deficiencies.

My older son would always sleep way more than other kids his age when he was little. At three years of age, he needed 15 hours of sleep a day; most kids get 10-12 hours at that age. People used to call me "the sleep nazi" because I was so committed to making sure that he got his naps; my life revolved around his sleep schedule. What those people didn't know is that there was hell to pay from a relentlessly crying child if I didn't ensure that schedule.

However, that all changed when a developmental psychiatrist advised us to take the railings off of his crib when he was three. After that, he was so stressed out about having his safe little nest taken away that he woke up five or six times a night, which meant that neither he nor I was getting to that deep, restful phase of sleep.

Hyperlexia

One of my sisters has seven children, and she has a theory that babies are either developing physically or they're developing mentally. This makes sense to me: given that my boys took so long to develop physically, their brains were busy developing mentally. By the time my older son turned two, he had a 1,000-word vocabulary and was saying things like "Mommy is sitting under the tree on a rock." My younger son had a similar vocabulary, and both taught themselves to read when they were three. I used to think this was a good thing, but Patricia Lemer, Chairman of the Board of Epidemic Answers, Co-Founder of Developmental Delay Resources, and author of *Outsmarting Autism: The Ultimate Guide to Management, Healing, and Prevention*, says it's a sign of uneven development, especially vision.

Low Body Temperature/Hypothyroidism

Check your child's basal body temperature before you get out of bed in the morning. If it's 97.8° Fahrenheit or under, he or she is very likely hypothyroid.

I always thought it was unusual that my sons typically had low body temperature, typically between 96.7° and 97.1° Fahrenheit. I remember asking the nurses at my former pediatricians' offices, and they seemed to think it was no big deal. It was a big deal because it's one of the most reliable indicators of hypothyroidism. The gist of low body temperature is that many biochemical reactions that are enzyme-dependent simply don't happen, leading to symptoms such as chronic sickness and fatigue.

In the case of children with neurodevelopmental disorders, the issue of hypothyroidism goes deeper because hypothyroidism is often one of the causes of these disorders. Dr. Raphael Kellman, a holistic endocrinologist in New York City presented at the AutismOne conference in 2012, saying that 75-80% of children with neurodevelopmental disorders are hypothyroid.[3]

3. Kellman, Raphael, MD, *The Thyroid-Autism Connection*, AutismOne Conference 2012, www.autismone.orgcontent/thyroid-autism-connection-2

Fatigue

Hypothyroidism is a common cause of fatigue, and roughly 80% of those who are hypothyroid also have some form of adrenal fatigue. Personally, I think the adrenal and thyroid issues are the most overlooked issues in this population, yet addressing them can have a huge beneficial impact on the health of these children. My boys had low energy and low stamina and would often get tired very easily.

Intolerance to Heat or Cold

An intolerance to heat or cold is actually a classic symptom of hypothyroidism, which I will discuss later in the book in relation to kids with SPD. I remember when my older son was younger that he would get upset if he were out in the heat for more than a few minutes.

UNDERSTANDING THE CAUSES

Have you ever wondered WHY there's such an epidemic of autism these days? Why is the rate now 1 in 68, when it was only 1 in 10,000 a couple of decades ago? Not only that, but WHY are there also epidemics of Sensory Processing Disorder, developmental delays, learning disabilities, ADHD, allergies, asthma, mood disorders, OCD, Lyme disease, autoimmune diseases, cancer and other chronic disorders?

There is no one single cause of autism or almost autism, Sensory Processing Disorder. Instead, these disorders are caused by what Beth Lambert, one of the founders of the Epidemic Answers non-profit for which I work, calls in her book, *A Compromised Generation: The Epidemic of Chronic Illness in America's Children*, the "perfect storm."

The perfect storm consists of toxicity, gut dysbiosis, immune dysregulation, nutritional deficiencies, hormonal imbalances and chronic inflammation. Unfortunately, what's not well known is that all of these factors can be passed from a mother to her fetus. In addition, children these days are exposed to unprecedented levels of stress, antibiotics, pharmaceuticals, poor diet, environmental toxins and excessive or improperly administered vaccines.

Toxicity

One of the main reasons for the epidemic of Sensory Processing Disorder as well as other children's chronic illnesses is the role of environmental toxicity. Dr. Phillip Landrigan and his team at the Mount Sinai Children's Environmental Health Center in New York City have documented the detrimental effects of certain toxins such as lead, mercury and flame retardants on the neurodevelopment of children. For example, epidemiologist Irva Hertz-Picciotto's research[1] says that a mom's proximity to car pollution raises her risk of having an autistic child.

Toxicity is one of the, if not THE, main reason why there is an epidemic of children's chronic illnesses today, such as autism, ADHD, allergies, asthma and autoimmune. As Jon Stewart said, "And that's just the A's". I include Sensory Processing Disorder, "almost autism," right in there with those disorders, as it has the same root causes as these disorders, as I'll explain.

You don't have to be living in a Superfund site to be exposed to toxins. These days, we're exposed to them through the air, water, food and personal-care products. Most people believe, like I used to, that surely this kind of information would be on the nightly TV news, but you won't find it there. Why? Follow the money. Look at the ads placed on TV and in newspapers and magazines. Pharmaceutical companies and big agricultural companies place the bulk of the ads, so those media outlets wouldn't say anything against those kinds of companies, lest their advertising funding disappear. They know who butters their bread.

In addition, most people think, like I used to, that if it's sold, it must be safe and surely all the governmental regulatory agencies like the FDA, CDC, USDA and EPA will protect us

1. http://www.eenews.net/stories/1059974806. Accessed August 28, 2014.

from harm. Not true. What most people don't know is that there is a revolving door between special-interest corporations with armies of lobbyists and these agencies.

For example, Michael Taylor is a former Vice President and lobbyist for Monsanto, a chemical company that brought us Agent Orange, saccharin, PCBs, polystyrene, DDT, dioxin, petroleum-based fertilizers, aspartame and Roundup® (glyphosate). Monsanto is now a leading supplier of genetically modified organisms (GMOs), which have been linked to rises in birth defects, asthma, allergies, autism and death, among other things. Michael Taylor was the FDA's Food Safety Czar when GMOs were allowed into the food supply without being tested; he is now Deputy Commissioner for Foods at the FDA. Do you see the conflict of interest here? Your family's health and safety are not in these agencies' best interests; money is, and this isn't an isolated case. The foxes are guarding the henhouse.

Passed from Mother to Child

I'm sorry to say that most people just don't know that babies are born pre-polluted. I didn't either, despite the fact that it was published by the Environmental Working Group (EWG) in 2005, the year my older son was born. In their landmark report, "Body Burden: The Pollution in Newborns,"[2] the EWG pointed out that an AVERAGE of 200 toxic chemicals were in the cordblood of newborns, meaning that there is only one place these could have come from: the mother. They found a total of over 280 carcinogens, heavy metals, endocrine disruptors, plastics, neurologically damaging pesticides and other nasties in these babies. It used to be thought that the barrier between the mother and the fetus would protect the fetus from toxins, but this report showed that it does not.

I remember telling our former pediatrician about the

2. http://www.ewg.org/research/body-burden-pollution-newborns. Accessed August 28, 2014.

shocking levels of heavy metals that I had discovered in myself and my sons. She said, "But you don't live in a toxic waste dump!" The point is, I don't think you have to anymore to be this toxic because we're all being exposed to these toxins on a daily basis, then unknowingly passing them onto our children, whose toxin load will accumulate over time, and they'll pass it on to their children. Research shows that toxins have an impact on the health of up to multiple generations later,[3] so if your great-great-great-great grandmother smoked cigarettes, the damaging effect of them affects your child's health.

Total Load Theory

Patricia Lemer talks about the total load theory in her new book, *Outsmarting Autism: The Ultimate Guide to Management, Healing, and Prevention.*[4] Basically, it's usually not one thing, unless it's a really big thing, that causes Sensory Processing Disorder or any other chronic disorder. Instead, it's an accumulation of a whole bunch of stressors that tip the scales in favor of the disorder, sort of like the straw that broke the camel's back.

According to a Swedish study,[5] a mother dumps 75% of her toxic load into her baby. Have you ever noticed that in most families with autism, ADHD, etc., that it's usually the older/oldest child who has the worst symptoms? That's because of the toxic load theory: they get more toxins than their siblings.

I believe my older son got the bigger dump because he was the first; there were more toxins for him to get from me. In addition, I was 39 years old when he was born, so that's 39

---

3. Gillette, Ross, et al, Sexually dimorphic effects of ancestral exposure to vinclozolin on stress reactivity in rats. *Endocrinology*, 2014; en.2014-1253 DOI: 10.1210/en.2014-1253

4. Lemer, Patricia S., *Outsmarting Autism: The Ultimate Guide to Management, Healing, and Prevention.* Tarentum, PA: Word Association, 2014, 9.

5. Darnerud PA, et.al. Polybrominated diphenyl ethers (PBDEs): Occurrence, Dietary Exposure, and Toxicology. *Environmental Health Perspectives*, 109, Supplement 1, 2001 Mar: 49-68.

years of accumulated toxins that he received. My younger son was born on my 41st birthday, and his heavy-metal toxicity was lower than his brother's but still substantially higher than average.

Bioaccumulation of Toxins

What's happening is that these toxins are bioaccumulating from one generation to the next. Do you remember how pregnant women are told to avoid large, fatty fish like tuna and swordfish because of the high levels of mercury they contain? These fish have that much mercury because it bioaccumulates: a tuna eats lots of smaller fish, which in turn eat lots of still-smaller fish. Mercury doesn't leave these fishes' bodies, so the levels continue to climb as you go further up the food chain, as in a tuna or swordfish. And people are at the very top of the food chain so all of those persistent pollutants like heavy metals, pesticides and plasticizers are accumulating inside of us. Both pesticides and plasticizers are known endocrine disruptors, and pesticides also damage the nervous system.

Other nasty toxins also bioaccumulate like perchlorate, polycyclic aromatic hydrocarbons (such as benzene and toluene), hexavalent chromium (the Erin Brockovich chemical), and tri-chloroethylene (TCE), which is now causing a huge epidemic of male breast cancer at Camp Lejeune Marine Corps Base. There's a documentary about this issue: *Semper Fi: Always Faithful.*

I believe this bioaccumulation of toxins from one generation to the next has reached a critical point and is the number one reason behind the growing epidemic of diseases, disorders and illnesses. Our babies are being born pre-polluted. The cards are stacked against them to begin with; they really don't stand much of a chance unless you detoxify them!

Sherry Rogers, MD, author of many books including *Detoxify or Die*, *The Cholesterol Hoax*, and *How to Cure Diabetes*, writes and lectures about how environmental toxins are continually overlooked by the medical profession as causes of disease. She should know because she recovered herself from Multiple Chemical Sensitivity and numerous other toxin-related illnesses and conditions. I really wish doctors and laypeople would read her books to gain an understanding of the nature of most chronic diseases and conditions: toxicity and nutritional deficiencies.

People are far more toxic than they realize, and the toxicity compounds from one generation to the next. In addition, some people are better at detoxifying than others, and this ability can vary depending on the ability to handle stress, the nutritional quality of a person's diet, exposure to toxins, and the use of antibiotics and pharmaceuticals.

Heavy Metals

According to the Mount Sinai Children's Environmental Health Center[6], heavy metals are one of the leading causes of neurodevelopmental damage. A recent study showed that autistic children have much higher levels of them than the general population[7] (that said, however, doesn't mean that the general population is free of heavy metals); the same holds true for children with Sensory Processing Disorder, ADD/ADHD and other neurodevelopmental disorders. These children have significantly higher levels of lead, thallium, tin, and tungsten, "toxic metals that can impair brain development and function, and also interfere with the normal functioning of other body organs and systems.[8]" The study also noted that "38-47% of the variation of autism severity was associated with the level of several toxic metals, with cadmium and mercury being the most strongly associated."

---

6. Landrigan, Philip J., et al, A Research Strategy to Discover the Environmental Causes of Autism and Neurodevelopmental Disabilities, *Environ Health Perspect.* Jul 2012; 120(7): a258–a260.
7. Adams, James B., et al, Toxicological Status of Children with Autism vs. Neurotypical Children and the Association with AutismSeverity. ***Biological Trace Element Research***, 2012; 151 (2): 171 DOI: 10.1007/s12011-012-9551-1
8. Ibid.

My Sons' Heavy-Metal Toxicity

After finding out that I had off-the-chart levels of heavy-metal toxicity, I immediately thought about my sons. Was it possible that I had passed any of this on to them? Could this be responsible for their Sensory Processing Disorder (SPD), asthma, allergies, eczema, acid reflux, and developmental delays? Would I finally find the common thread that I had been looking for all along that tied all of these conditions together? Yes, unfortunately.

After finding out about my toxicity, I had both sons tested with a heavy-metal hair test from Doctor's Data because it's not invasive. My older son was in the 97th percentile for heavy-metal toxicity; my younger at the 90th. That means that my older son had more heavy metals in him than 97% of people in the reference group, which contains roughly 40,000 people.

Heavy Metal	**Reference Range (µg/g)**	**Older Son (µg/g)**	**Younger Son (µg/g)**
Aluminum	**<8.000**	**16.000**	**13.000**
Antimony	**<0.066**	**0.110**	**0.210**
Arsenic	<0.080	0.047	**0.098**
Barium	<0.500	**0.830**	0.360
Beryllium	<0.020	<0.010	<0.010
Bismuth	<2.000	0.078	0.100
Cadmium	**<0.070**	**0.110**	0.041
Lead	**<1.000**	**2.100**	0.970
Mercury	**<0.400**	**0.530**	**0.500**
Nickel	**<0.200**	**0.330**	0.080
Platinum	<0.005	<0.003	<0.003

Silver	**<0.200**	**0.530**	**0.260**
Thallium	<0.002	<0.001	<0.001
Thorium	<0.002	0.001	**0.003**
Tin	**<0.300**	**0.810**	**0.350**
Titanium	<1.000	0.630	0.770
Uranium	<0.060	0.026	0.011

My older son had elevated levels of aluminum, antimony, barium, cadmium, lead, mercury, nickel, silver and tin, while my younger son's levels of aluminum, antimony, arsenic, mercury, silver, thorium and tin were higher than normal.

I believe the high levels of aluminum, lead and mercury in them (they were ages three and four when I had them tested) were responsible for their Sensory Processing Disorder, as these metals are known neurotoxins that damage the nervous system, and SPD is a nervous-system disorder.

Heavy Metal Sources

You may be wondering, as I was, how the heck my sons got so polluted. Guess what? They got it from me. You read that right. I really felt sick to my stomach when I realized that I had unknowingly passed these toxins on to my boys. And then I got angry, really angry. Why hadn't I been warned? Why don't doctors know about this?

The truth is that most pediatricians and other doctors have not been trained in medical school to look for environmental causes of illness, despite the growing preponderance of evidence and the growing epidemic of autoimmune diseases. If you want the real answers to these questions, you have to do your own research and look outside the narrow viewpoint of conventional Western medicine.

Obviously, I can only theorize as to the sources of heavy metals for myself and for my children because we are not lab rats in a controlled-environment experiment, and I can't "prove" how these heavy metals got inside of me.

I grew up in east Tennessee, in the foothills of the Smoky Mountains (cue banjo music now, I know). In our town, there was a coal-fired power plant. Did you know that coal is laden with heavy metals? In fact, there was an environmental disaster a few years ago in the town where I went to high school because a dike of the retention pond that holds all of the sludgy waste from the smokestacks broke and all that sludgy waste dumped into the river for miles, polluting the beautiful lakes and rivers around it. Test results showed significantly elevated levels of toxic metals including arsenic, copper, barium, cadmium, chromium, lead, mercury, nickel, and thallium in samples of the slurry and river water. Even though I was no longer living in the town when this disaster happened, I had grown up breathing this nasty air for years and the metals had seeped into the groundwater that I drank on a daily basis.

Later, I lived in Baton Rouge for four years and in New Orleans for 10 years, well before my boys were born. The Mississippi River in those parts is called "Cancer Alley" because of all the oil refineries along the river that dump waste into the water. There's a pretty good chance that there are heavy metals in the water, too, I bet, in addition to all the carcinogenic petroleum byproducts in there. Even though I drank mostly bottled spring water, I was still cooking, cleaning and bathing in the tap water.

I moved to New York City from New Orleans and lived there for a good five years after 9/11, breathing in all those toxic fumes from the Twin Towers for months after they fell; my older son was born in 2005. As part of the 10th anniversary of 9/11, *Scientific American* published an article called, "What Was in the World Trade Center Plume?"[9] The author found that people living and working in New York City were exposed to lead, mercury, tungsten and other heavy metals, record levels of dioxins, PCBs, polycyclic aromatic

---

9. Biello, David. "What Was in the World Trade Center Plume?" *Scientific American*, Sep. 7, 2011.

hydrocarbons and asbestos for the more than three months that the World Trade Center fires smoldered.

Mercury

The symptoms of mercury toxicity mimics the symptoms of autism, writes Kenneth Bock MD in *Healing the New Childhood Epidemics: Autism, ADHD, Asthma, and Allergies.*[10] Some of the common symptoms are:

- Clumsiness
- Slow physical development
- Sound sensitivity
- Touch avoidance
- Inattentiveness
- Delayed speech/loss of ability to speak
- Poor cognitive processing
- Hypotonia
- Dermatitis
- Allergies
- Asthma
- Autoimmune disorder

In addition, Dr. Russell Blaylock in *Health and Nutrition Secrets That Can Save Your Life*, writes that some additional symptoms of mercury poisoning are:

- Personality changes
- Unusual irritability
- Timidity or shyness
- Insomnia
- Apathy
- Impaired concentration[11]

---

10. Bock, Kenneth, MD. *Healing the New Childhood Epidemics: Autism, ADHD, Asthma, and Allergies*. New York, NY: Ballantine Books, 2008, 54-55.
11. Blaylock, Russell, MD. *Health and Nutrition Secrets That Can Save Your Life.* Albuquerque, NM: Health Press, 2006, 41.

Does this sound like your SPD child? I bet it does. Dan Olmsted and Mark Blaxill say in *The Age of Autism: Mercury, Medicine, and a Man-Made Epidemic* that one in six children is born with blood levels of mercury high enough to cause a neurodevelopmental disorder later on in life.[12] Sickening.

Mercury is perhaps the most insidious of the heavy metals. It binds with and inactivates glutathione, the body's principal protection antioxidant, thereby preventing the body from getting rid of it. Because of this, it greatly increases inflammation, what's known as free-radical production or lipid peroxidation in medical parlance.

Mercury also attaches to macrophages, a type of white blood cell, thereby inhibiting the body's ability to rid itself of the yeast *Candida albicans*. Because of this, a child whose body is laden with mercury is more susceptible to infection and more likely to be chronically sick.

"Silver" fillings in your mouth are actually 50% mercury. The mercury when it's transported to and from your dentist's office has to be labeled "hazardous waste." Why is it suddenly not hazardous waste just because it's in your mouth? There's a famous video on the IAOMT (the International Academy of Oral Medicine and Toxicology) website[13] that shows "smoking teeth," i.e., mercury vapor off-gassing from a mercury filling. Guess where that mercury goes to? That's right – your body! It goes there faster if you're eating or drinking something hot. My advice: get your "silver" fillings removed by an IAOMT dentist who is specially trained to remove them without harming you or him/herself and staff. I believe mercury amalgams are one of the greatest environmental threats, and the problem worsens with each generation because of bio-accumulation.[14] If you had "silver" fillings in your mouth

12. Olmsted, Dan and Blaxill, Mark, *The Age of Autism: Mercury, Medicine, and a Man-Made Epidemic.* New York, NY: Thomas Dunne Books, 2010, ii.
13. http://library.iaomt.org/document/smoking-teeth-poison-gas. Accessed August 28, 2014.
14. Palkovicova L et al, Maternal amalgam dental fillings as the source of mercury exposure in developing fetus and newborn, *J Expo Sci Environ Epidemiol.* 2008 May;18(3):326-31.

before or during the time when you were pregnant with your child, there's a good chance that the mercury in those fillings off-gassed into your body and was passed onto your child.

Large fish, such as large tuna, sharks and swordfish, contain some of the highest amounts of mercury of seafood. All that sushi I had eaten most likely contained mercury! Actor Jeremy Piven and actresses Hillary Swank and Daphne Zuniga all reportedly suffered from mercury poisoning from eating too much tuna.

Many flu vaccines contain 25 micrograms of mercury in the form of thimerosal,[15] as does a tetanus vaccine and the multi-dose version of the meningococcal vaccine.[16] In addition, even though thimerosal isn't listed as an ingredient on the insert of many vaccines, it is still there because it's used in the manufacturing process. The FDA ruled that because it is a preservative, it doesn't have to be listed as an ingredient, so many vaccines that should have only trace amounts of it actually have far greater levels.[17]

Mercury is used to produce food additives such as citric acid, sodium benzoate and high-fructose corn syrup (HFCS). "The production process can create a mercury level of 0.005-0.57 micrograms of mercury per gram of HFCS," writes Sherry Rogers, MD. Thus, with the average American consuming 50 grams of HFCS per day, that's the "*equivalent of having two teeth filled with mercury amalgam every single day of your life.*" [18]

Mercury is still found in many brands of mascara[19], and it's also found in fluorescent light bulbs.

---

15. Kennedy, Robert F., Jr., Editor, *Thimerosal: Let the Science Speak* . New York, NY: Skyhorse Publishing, 2014, xxx.
16. http://www.vaccinesafety.edu/thi-table.htm. Accessed September 11, 2014.
17. http://vaxtruth.org/2011/09/the-flu-vaccine-what-your-doctor-wont-tell-you-or-probably-doesnt-even-know/. Accessed September 11, 2014.
18. Rogers, Sherry, MD, *Total Wellness Newsletter*, February 2014, 3.
19. http://www.scientificamerican.com/article/in-the-public-eye-mascara-exempt-from-mercury-treaty/. Accessed September 11, 2014.

Lead

Lead is a neurotoxin, and children with elevated lead levels are more likely to be hyperactive and impulsive; elevated levels of lead are often found in children with ADHD.[20]

Where does lead come from? It's not like Americans use leaded gas anymore. For starters, lead is often found in old houses built before 1978, when lead-based paint was banned. The problem is that homeowners that renovate their old houses can expose themselves and their children to lead when sanding and stripping off old paint; proper precautions must be taken. Really old houses, like the ones in which I lived in New Orleans, also have thick, lead-based glass in the window panes, which look a little warped when you look through them.

Old neighborhoods also have old lead-based pipes within them and lead pipes leading up to them from the city's water supply. Lead easily leaches out of these old pipes and into the tap water.

Lead and tin are both used in ceramic glazes, and the dishes I'd been using for years had become scratched and chipped, easily letting the heavy metals out. Lead is used in crystal glasses and dishes. Wine lovers prefer these special glasses because it makes the wine taste a little sweeter. I think we need to remember that it was the use of lead in goblets and dishes that led to the fall of the Roman Empire. Everyone went "plumb" crazy; the Latin word for lead is "plumbum".

The isotope of radioactive thorium that is used in medical testing is Th-232, which eventually decays to lead. It's typically used as a coating for tungsten in incandescent light bulbs.

Some types of cosmetics still contain lead (usually red lipsticks), as the Environmental Working Group wrote about in their article, "I'll take my lipstick unleaded, please".[21]

In addition, honey that isn't locally produced typically

---

20. Nigg, Joel, Attention-Deficit/Hyperactivity Disorder: Endophenotypes, Structure, and Etiological Pathways. *Current Directions in Psychological Science,* February, 2010

21. http://www.ewg.org/kid-safe-chemicals-act-blog/2009/09/ill-take-my-lipstick-unleaded-please/. Accessed August 30, 2014.

comes from overseas. Chinese honey is stored in lead containers, and the lead leaches into the honey[22], as was discussed in *Food Safety News.* Even if you eat locally produced honey, you're probably unknowingly consuming lead-tainted honey if you're eating processed foods containing honey like honey-flavored cereals.

Cadmium

Prenatal exposure to cadmium, even at low levels, can have long-lasting effects on children's IQ, as it is a neurotoxin.[23] Cadmium is found in NiCad batteries, plastics, car exhaust and fertilizers. Cadmium can also be found in cheap jewelry, especially if it's from China, and most products are made in China these days. The *San Francisco Chronicle*, in an article entitled, "Toxic cadmium common in China's cheap jewelry," wrote that "Barred from using lead in children's jewelry because of its toxicity, some Chinese manufacturers have been substituting the more dangerous heavy metal cadmium."[24]

Cigarette smoke, even if it's secondhand, contains cadmium, and, "for each pack of cigarettes smoked, a person can absorb an additional 1-3 mcg of cadmium over what is taken in from other sources in their daily life."[25] Although I didn't smoke, my mother smoked three packs of cigarettes a day when I was growing up; after watching *Mad Men*, I'm thinking it was the norm back then.

Dr. Russell Blaylock, in *Health and Nutrition Secrets That Can Change Your Life,* writes that, "Clear plastic wrap used to

---

22. http://www.foodsafetynews.com/2011/08/honey-laundering/#.VAIbXEh8HYs. Accessed August 30, 2014.
23. Kippler M, et al, Early-Life cadmium exposure and child development in 5-year-old girls and boys: a Cohort study in rural Bangladesh. *Environmental Health Perspectives* http://dx.doi.org/10.1289/ehp.1104431.
24. http://www.sfgate.com/world/article/Toxic-cadmium-common-in-China-s-cheap-jewelry-3276017.php. Accessed August 30, 2014.
25. http://quitsmoking.about.com/od/chemicalsinsmoke/p/cadmium.htm. Accessed August 30, 2014.

cover dishes also contains cadmium and should not be microwaved or in any way heated. It should be safe in the refrigerator."[26] I'm not sure if this includes all those plastic covers on the Lean Cuisine, Weight Watcher's and Amy's Kitchen meals I ate for many years.

Drinking water is another source of cadmium. Even if levels are low in the water itself, both plastic (PVC) and metal pipes typically contain cadmium as well as lead[27].

Aluminum

Aluminum is another neurotoxin that is commonly found in children with ADHD[28], as well as other neurodevelopmental disorders such as Sensory Processing Disorder and autism. Aluminum is, of course, commonly found in aluminum cans, foil, pots and pans, but it's also found in many anti-perspirants.

Heather Fraser wrote in *The Peanut Allergy Epidemic: What's Causing It and How to Stop It,* that aluminum and other adjuvants are "the immunologists' dirty little secret" because they are used in vaccines to over-excite the immune system.[29] Despite the removal of mercury in the form of thimerosal from most vaccines, most parents don't know about the damaging effects of aluminum that are in a number of vaccines given to their children, as Joseph Mercola, DO, wrote about in the article, "Aluminum, the Neurotoxin Far Worse Than Mercury…[30]

---

26. Blaylock, Russell, MD. *Health and Nutrition Secrets That Can Save Your Life.* Albuquerque, NM: Health Press, 2006,, 136.
27. http://www.everydayexposures.com/toxins/toxic-metals/cadmium. Accessed August 30, 2014.
28. Nicolescu R, et al, Environmental exposure to lead, but not other neurotoxic metals, relates to core elements of ADHD in Romanian children: performance and questionnaire data, *Environ Res.* 2010 Jul;110(5):476-83. doi: 10.1016/j.envres.2010.04.002.
29. Fraser, H. *The Peanut Allergy Epidemic: What's Causing It and How to Stop It.* New York, NY: Skyhorse Publishing, 2011, 104.
30. http://articles.mercola.com/sites/articles/archive/2011/09/21/could-this-be-the-most-dangerous-aspect-of-vaccines.aspx. Accessed August 30, 2014.

Look up in the sky. Those aren't old-fashioned contrails hazing up our skies anymore. Contrails disappear pretty quickly. Those are geoengineering chemtrails filled with heavy metals like aluminum and barium that fall on you and me, and they're used for climate control. Keep an eye on the sky next time you see white streaks across it; within minutes, they'll spread out into feathery clouds, and within an hour or two, the sky will be hazy. Don't believe me? Even the *Washington Post* knows about it, as they published in the article, "Geoengineering is the answer to climate change. Unless it isn't."[31]

Arsenic

Chicken, if it's not organic, contains arsenic, as part of an anti-fungal used on the chicken feed. What's worse is that "arsenic in poultry manure is rapidly converted into an inorganic form that is highly water soluble and capable of moving into surface and ground water."[32] Given that chickens and rice are raised in many of the same geographical areas, it's no coincidence that arsenic from chicken poop shows up in rice-growing areas.[33]

Food & Water Watch discovered a few years ago that the amount of arsenic in apple juice was exceedingly high in major brands such as Mott's, which had levels of 55 parts per billion. The EPA's limit on arsenic in well water is 10 parts per billion. The U.S. imports about 70% of its apple juice from China, where food safety and inspection is unimpressive.[34]

---

31. http://www.washingtonpost.com/national/health-science/geoengineering-is-the-answer-to-climate-change-unless-it-isnt/2012/11/05/aef1c418-073d-11e2-858a-5311df86ab04_story.html. Accessed August 30, 2014.
32. http://www.livablefutureblog.com/2010/06/the-hidden-hazard-of-poultry-litter-pelletization. Accessed September 11, 2014.
33. http://www.motherjones.com/tom-philpott/2012/09/waiter-theres-arsenic-my-rice. Accessed September 11, 2014.
34. http://www.foodsafetynews.com/2011/07/arsenic-laced-apple-juice-flowing-from-china/#.VBGcF0h8HYs. Accessed September 11, 2014.

Arsenic can also come from well water, pressure-treated wood, refineries and insecticides.

Vaccinations

I realize the issue of vaccinations is an uncomfortable one for many parents to think about. It's a very polarizing subject, I get that, but if you believe that the whole issue of vaccine injury has been laid to rest, you're not thinking and you're not doing your research. Instead, what you typically see or hear in the media is that the whole issue was settled years ago. It hasn't been. This information is told to us by reporters who are not investigating the facts because, if they were researching, they would have something else entirely to say. You're not likely to hear about this on the evening news because Big Pharma pays for most of the ads. Follow the money. Those reporters know who butters their bread.

If you repeat a lie often enough, people will believe it. As Carl Sagan wrote, "One of the saddest lessons of history is this: If we've been bamboozled long enough, we tend to reject any evidence of the bamboozle. We're no longer interested in finding out the truth. The bamboozle has captured us. It's simply too painful to acknowledge, even to ourselves, that we've been taken. Once you give a charlatan power over you, you almost never get it back."[35]

As an example of how long the Center for Disease Control (CDC) has known about the link between vaccination and autism, a whistleblower, William Thompson – a researcher for the CDC, came forward on August 27, 2014 saying that the CDC covered up the link between the MMR vaccine and autism since at least 2004, when data was purposefully omitted from a peer-reviewed study showing a 2.4x increased risk of autism in African American males receiving the MMR vaccine before the age of 36 months. A two-fold increase in risk is

35. Sagan, C., *The Demon-Haunted World: Science as a Candle in the Dark.* New York, NY: Ballantine, 1996, 241.

sufficient in a court of law to prove causation. THIS IS FRAUD, and I am angry!

Thompson released a statement through his attorneys, saying:

> I regret that my coauthors and I omitted statistically significant information in our 2004 article published in the journal *Pediatrics*. The omitted data suggested that African American males who received the MMR vaccine before age 36 months were at increased risk for autism. Decisions were made regarding which findings to report after the data were collected, and I believe that the final study protocol was not followed.[36]

As of the writing of this book, no large media service has looked into this, except to briefly speak about the whistleblower and then quickly repeat the party line that vaccines are safe. However, Representative Bill Posey from Florida is calling for a congressional investigation into the CDC's cover-up, as his office likely has 100,000 documents turned over to him by the whistleblower, William Thompson.

There are actually dozens of peer-reviewed medical research studies proving vaccine injury. For example, a newly published study concludes that "rising autistic prevalence is directly related to vaccines manufactured utilizing human fetal cells." It's an epidemiological study that says that change points in the rate of autism (in the U.S., that's 1980.9, 1988.4 and 1996) "corresponded to introduction of or increased doses of human fetal cell line-manufactured vaccines, while no relationship was found between paternal age or *Diagnostic and Statistical Manual (DSM)* revisions and autistic disorder diagnosis."[37] Fetal cells come from **aborted human fetuses**

---

36. http://www.morganverkamp.com/august-27-2014-press-release-statement-of-william-w-thompson-ph-d-regarding-the-2004-article-examining-the-possibility-of-a-relationship-between-mmr-vaccine-and-autism/. Accessed September 9, 2014.

37. Deisher, Theresa A., Impact of environmental factors on the prevalence of autistic disorder after 1979, *Journal of Public Health and Epidemiology*, ol.6(9),

and are used in the MMR, chickenpox, smallpox, rabies and hepatitis A vaccines. If that isn't enough to make you throw up, I don't what is.

In addition to containing tissue from aborted human fetuses, vaccines also may contain a mix of:

- **Formaldehyde:** A carcinogen used for embalming corpses.
- **Aluminum:** A heavy metal that is a known neurotoxin.
- **Mercury:** Another heavy metal that is also a known neurotoxin. There are 25 mcg of mercury in the average flu shot, and the EPA safety limit is 5 micrograms.
- **Phenoxyethanol:** A chemical that is highly toxic to the nervous system, kidneys, and liver.
- **Polysorbate 80:** An emulsifier and excipient linked to anaphylactic shock.
- **Bovine cow serum:** Cow skin extract linked to autoimmune disorders.
- **MSG:** A known neurotoxin that causes brain cell death.

Here are some things to consider when doing your research about vaccine safety:

- As an example, the vaccine insert on the DTaP shot specifically states that autism, seizures, death, anaphylactic shock and SIDS are risks. Do you ever read those inserts? I never did. I didn't even know they existed until after my sons were fully vaccinated. If you don't believe me, take a look here at the package insert.

September 2014, p. 271.

Page 11 of 13

In the German case-control study and US open-label safety study in which 14,971 infants received Tripedia vaccine, 13 deaths in Tripedia vaccine recipients were reported. Causes of deaths included seven SIDS, and one of each of the following: enteritis, Leigh Syndrome, adrenogenital syndrome, cardiac arrest, motor vehicle accident, and accidental drowning. All of these events occurred more than two weeks post immunization.[2] The rate of SIDS observed in the German case-control study was 0.4/1,000 vaccinated infants. The rate of SIDS observed in the US open-label safety study was 0.8/1,000 vaccinated infants and the reported rate of SIDS in the US from 1985-1991 was 1.5/1,000 live births.[34] By chance alone, some cases of SIDS can be expected to follow receipt of whole-cell pertussis DTP[35] or DTaP vaccines.

Additional Adverse Reactions:

- As with other aluminum-containing vaccines, a nodule may be palpable at the injection sites for several weeks. Sterile abscess formation at the site of injection has been reported.[3,36]
- Rarely, an anaphylactic reaction (ie, hives, swelling of the mouth, difficulty breathing, hypotension, or shock) has been reported after receiving preparations containing diphtheria, tetanus, and/or pertussis antigens.[3]
- Arthus-type hypersensitivity reactions, characterized by severe local reactions (generally starting 2-8 hours after an injection), may follow receipt of tetanus toxoid.
- A few cases of peripheral mononeuropathy and of cranial mononeuropathy have been reported following tetanus toxoid administration, although available evidence is inadequate to accept or reject a causal relation.[37]
- A review by the Institute of Medicine (IOM) found evidence for a causal relationship between tetanus toxoid and both brachial neuritis and Guillain-Barré syndrome.[37]
- A few cases of demyelinating diseases of the CNS have been reported following some tetanus toxoid-containing vaccines or tetanus and diphtheria toxoid-containing vaccines, although the IOM concluded that the evidence was inadequate to accept or reject a causal relationship.[37]

Adverse events reported during post-approval use of Tripedia vaccine include idiopathic thrombocytopenic purpura, SIDS, anaphylactic reaction, cellulitis, autism, convulsion/grand mal convulsion, encephalopathy, hypotonia, neuropathy, somnolence and apnea. Events were included in this list because of the seriousness or frequency of reporting. Because these events are reported voluntarily from a population of uncertain size, it is not always possible to reliably estimate their frequencies or to establish a causal relationship to components of Tripedia vaccine.[2]

SOURCE: Sanofi Pasteur Inc.: Package insert for Diphtheria and Tetanus Toxoids and Acellular Pertussis Vaccine Adsorbed Tripedia®

- Children today receive at least 69 doses of vaccines by the time they are 18, roughly 4 times the level kids received 30+ years ago, and new vaccines are constantly introduced.
- Vaccines have never been tested for safety in the U.S. by the CDC. There has never been a double-blind study between vaccinated and unvaccinated children in the U.S. by the CDC.
- There has never been a study in the U.S. by the CDC confirming the safety of giving multiple shots in one day.
- Giving Tylenol® to your baby on the day of vaccination is the worst thing you can do because it lowers the amount of glutathione – the body's master antioxidant – in the body. Glutathione is necessary for your child's body to detoxify from toxins in vaccines and other sources.
- The vaccine watch organization Sanevax reports over 150 deaths from the Gardasil® vaccine,[38] and, even if people

38. http://www.greenmedinfo.com/blog/hpv-vaccines-unnecessary-and-

don't die from it, it can be highly debilitating by causing pain, paralysis, MS, seizures, encephalitis and fatigue as shown in the documentary, *The Greater Good.*

- Dr. Julie Gerberding was the head of the CDC from 2002 to 2009 and was in charge of vaccine/autism research. She now leads the vaccine division for Merck, the maker of the very vaccine most of the research was about. As you'll notice throughout this book, there is a revolving door between government agencies such as the CDC, FDA and USDA – agencies supposedly there to protect our health – and the industries that they are charged to regulate.
- As of the U.S. government's fiscal year 2014, $3.0 billion has been paid out to plaintiffs from the national Vaccine Injury Compensation Program (VICP) – also known as vaccine court.[39] The fund was created by the Reagan administration after President Reagan signed the National Childhood Vaccine Injury Act in 1988, which protected vaccine manufacturers from being sued for damages created by their vaccines. Because vaccine court is a no-fault alternative to the tort system, vaccine manufacturers gained free rein to introduce whatever they wanted to without penalty. Thus began increased dosage and multiple vaccinations. In 1985, seven vaccines were given to children. By 2007, the number had grown to 37, and today it's at least 69. Beginning in 1993, multiple vaccinations were given in a single needle. To understand how vaccine court is tilted in Big Pharma's favor, I highly recommend the 5-minute YouTube video narrated by Rob Schneider, "Do Vaccines Cause Autism?"[40]

I urge you to research this subject for yourself. I used to turn a blind eye to it and assume that whatever the pediatrician

---

lethal. Accessed September 10, 2014.
39. http://www.hrsa.gov/vaccinecompensation/statisticsreport.pdf. Accessed September 10, 2014.
40. https://www.youtube.com/watch?v=xv_IaLHwgAQ. Accessed September 10, 2014.

gave my children was safe. Your child's health can't afford the luxury of ignorant bliss anymore, unfortunately, so here are some starting points for you to learn more:

- National Vaccine Information Center: www.nvic.org
- *Vaccine Epidemic: How Corporate Greed, Biased Science, and Coercive Government Threaten Our Human Rights, Our Health, and Our Children,* by Louise Kuo Habakus
- *The Vaccine Book: Making the Right Decision for Your Child (Sears Parenting Library)* by Robert W. Sears, MD, FAAP
- *The Peanut Allergy Epidemic: What's Causing It and How to Stop It* by Heather Fraser. Heather explains how it's the combination of peanut oil and adjuvants, "the immunologists' dirty little secret", that is causing the alarming rise in peanut allergies.[41] When I was a kid, no one I knew had allergies, peanut allergies, asthma, Sensory Processing Disorder or autism. Now over half of American children have some form of chronic illness. It's the new normal.
- *A Shot in the Dark* by Harris L. Coulter and Barbara Loe Fisher
- *What Your Doctor May Not Tell You About Your Children's Vaccinations* by Stephanie F. Cave, MD
- SaneVax, Inc.: www.sanevax.org
- *Thimerosal: Let the Science Speak: The Evidence Supporting the Immediate Removal of Mercury – a Known Neurotoxin – from Vaccines*, Robert F. Kennedy, Jr., Editor
- VaxTruth: www.vaxtruth.org

I can't sit idly by and say nothing about the dangers of vaccines. In fact, too many of my friends and clients have children that regressed into autism after vaccination. Some of them have uploaded their child's vaccine-injury story onto YouTube, and you can view hundreds of these heartbreaking

41. Fraser, H.,*The Peanut Allergy Epidemic: What's Causing It and How to Stop It.* New York, NY: Skyhorse Publishing, 2011, 104.

stories by typing in "#hearthiswell" in the YouTube search bar. You can also read some of their stories in *The Thinking Moms' Revolution: Autism beyond the Spectrum: Inspiring True Stories from Parents Fighting to Rescue Their Children* and *Evolution of a Revolution: From Hope to Healing.*

Here's my theory on vaccinations: I believe they are sometimes the last straw to break the poor child's "back" (immune system). Kids today are born so pre-polluted that vaccines and their adjuvants can sometimes be the external factors that put their immune systems into overdrive. In addition, a child who has a cold, ear infections or any kind of chronic condition such as allergies, eczema, chronic constipation and asthma should not be vaccinated because it means their immune system is compromised. Unfortunately, most pediatricians don't look for these soft signs.

Pharmaceuticals

As Sherry Rogers, MD, so often says, "drugs work by simply poisoning a pathway" and "the sick get sicker quicker" when they take pharmaceuticals; that's why there are so many nasty side effects to taking them. Pharmaceuticals put a tremendous amount of strain on the already toxic, overloaded liver of your SPD child.

Tylenol®

Tylenol®, also known as acetaminophen and paracetamol, is toxic to the liver, which is why the FDA is considering pulling it from the shelves. According to the Mayo Clinic, taking too much Tylenol® is the leading cause of acute liver failure.[42] Studies have shown that use of it is correlated with increased neurodevelopmental damage.[43, 44] Dr. William

---

42. http://www.mayoclinic.org/diseases-conditions/liver-failure/basics/causes/con-20030966. Accessed September 25, 2014.
43. Brandlistuen RE, Prenatal paracetamol exposure and child

Shaw of the Great Plains Laboratory has a highly detailed presentation about it on Vimeo entitled, "Increased Acetaminophen Use Appears to Be the Major Cause of Autism".[45] Dr. Shaw also published his research findings in the *Journal of Restorative Medicine* where he wrote that "Compared with controls, children aged 1–5 years with autism were eight times more likely to have become unwell after the MMR vaccine, and were six times more likely to have taken acetaminophen. Children with autism who regressed in development were four times more likely to have taken acetaminophen after the vaccine." [46]

Dr. Shaw points out that Cuba – a country where vaccines are mandatory – has an autism incidence of rate of 0.00168% versus the current rate of 1.5% in America. The practice of prescribing Tylenol® is very uncommon in Cuba, as it's only available by prescription and is not used prophylactically in combination with vaccines. What's sickening is that researchers have known about the damage that Tylenol® does since at least 1977, when an FDA advisory panel ensured that a warning about the drug's toxicity to the liver was placed on the label. Not coincidentally, a study concluded, there was a drop in the autism rate.[47]

Some of the worst pieces of advice we get from the doctor are: "Give Tylenol® right before or after shots" and "Give Tylenol® or ibuprofen to bring a fever down." Here's why:

---

neurodevelopment: a sibling-controlled cohort study, *Int J Epidemiol.* 2013 Dec;42(6):1702-13

44. Seneff, S., et al, Empirical Data Confirm Autism Symptoms Related to Aluminum and Acetaminophen Exposure, *Entropy* 2012, 14(11), 2227-2253.

45. http://vimeo.com/78937547. Accessed September 10, 2014.

46. Shaw, W. Ground-breaking Theory Proposes Acetaminophen Use Linked to Autism, *Journal of Restorative Medicine*, Volume 2, Number 1, October 2013 , pp. 14-29(16).

47. Schultz S.T., et al, Acetaminophen (paracetamol) use, measles-mumps rubella vaccination, and autistic disorder: The results of a parent survey. *Autism.* 2008;12(3):293–307.

- First of all, giving Tylenol® reduces glutathione, the body's master antioxidant, which is needed to detoxify. Giving Tylenol® right before or after shots ties your child's immune system's hands behind its back, leaving your child very vulnerable to the adjuvants in the vaccine. Just so you know, ibuprofen isn't any better because it damages the linings of the gut and stomach.
- Second of all, fever is not a bad thing, unless it gets really high. My personal cutoff is 102° Fahrenheit, but you should discuss this with your pediatrician to determine what's right for your child. I won't give anything to my kids with a fever like this. A fever is the body's way of fighting off infection, and if you teach the immune system it doesn't need to work, it won't when it really needs to.

Acid-Reflux Medication

Prevacid® and other proton-pump inhibitors (PPI) such as Nexium®, Zantac®, Prilosec® and omeprazole are not doing your child favor by turning down the stomach acid; neither are acid blockers such as Tums®. Your child NEEDS stomach acid for a few reasons:

- The gastrointestinal tract is the first line of defense against viruses, bacteria and parasites. The less stomach acid your child has, the less they're able to fight off those bugs and the more they'll get sick. By prescribing acid-reflux medication, doctors are putting their patients at a higher risk for infections like pneumonia and gastroenteritis, as well as getting more colds and stomach bugs. In addition, by taking acid-reflux drugs, your child is more likely to get sick more often because their immune system can't fight off these offenders. It also makes the rest of the gastrointestinal tract susceptible to bacterial overgrowth.[48]

48. Lombardo, L., Increased incidence of small intestinal bacterial overgrowth during proton pump inhibitor therapy, *Clin Gastroenterol Hepatol.*

- Stomach acid aids in the absorption of critical nutrients, such as iron, magnesium, calcium and vitamin B_{12}.[49] Without enough stomach acid, your child can become anemic, and two common types of anemia, iron-deficiency anemia and pernicious anemia – a type of anemia caused by a vitamin B_{12} deficiency – are often found in SPD children. In fact, in the book *Could It Be B_{12}? An Epidemic of Misdiagnoses*, authors Sally Pacholok and Jeffrey Stuart discuss how people who have had gastric bypass surgery (stomach stapling or bands) WILL develop a dangerous B_{12} deficiency because they no longer have enough stomach acid to help absorb it. Long-term B_{12} deficiency can lead to severe neurological damage and its symptoms can mimic autism and other illnesses.
- Stomach acid is crucial for the breakdown of proteins into their constituent amino acids. SPD children may be deficient in amino acids such as tryptophan, GABA, glycine, cysteine and carnitine.

Is it worth it for your child to take acid-reflux medication? I don't think so, and I can tell you that, as a mom, after I found out how truly dangerous these drugs are, I was upset at the doctors – pediatricians, allergists and gastroenterologists – who prescribed them to my boys for their acid reflux without discovering the real source of their reflux: a dairy sensitivity and gut dysbiosis.

Miralax® and Other Synthetic Laxatives

Many children with Sensory Processing Disorder typically have chronic constipation, but if your child is taking Miralax® or any other laxative that contains polyethylene glycol, they are essentially ingesting antifreeze, which is ethylene glycol.

2010 Jun;8(6):504-8.

49. Hassall, E., Over-prescription of acid-suppressing medications in infants: how it came about, why it's wrong, and what to do about it, *J Pediatr.* 2012 Feb;160(2):193-8.

Chemically speaking, polyethylene glycol is made from stringing ethylene glycols together. Many parents continue to give it to their children for constipation, perhaps because they are unaware of the FDA's safety alert in December 2011 that Miralax® and its clones are neurotoxins.[50] Because polyethylene glycol blocks nutrient absorption, it may lead to the onset of autism in a toddler with severe iron or iodine deficiency.[51]

Be careful of its pseudonym "Carbowax Sentry," which shows up in chewing gum, energy drinks, toothpastes, lotions, soaps and shampoos. Polyethylene glycol is also an excellent toilet-bowl cleaner, so maybe it should just be used for that.

If your child suffers from constipation, I'll be discussing what to do about that later in the book when I talk about "Check the Poop." Unfortunately, most pediatricians don't realize it can happen due to food sensitivities and gut dysbiosis, which I will also be explaining later in the book.

Cortisone and Other Steroids

Children with SPD often have comorbid conditions such as eczema and asthma, which are often treated with steroids to reduce swelling and inflammation that cause rashes, itching and/or trouble breathing. The problem is that steroids quickly damage the immune system and lead to gut dysbiosis. In the case of my older son's eczema, which he had since he was a tiny baby, pediatricians always told me to "just put a little cortisone cream on it." What they didn't tell me is that doing so drives the disease process deeper into the body and into the lungs, another route of elimination, and often leads to the development of asthma later. My older son developed life-threatening asthma at the age of four and was then treated with

---

50. http://www.fda.gov/Drugs/GuidanceComplianceRegulatory Information/Surveillance/AdverseDrugEffects/ucm295585.htm. Accessed September 10, 2014.

51. www.gutsense.org/gutsense/the-role-of-miralax-laxative-in-autism-dementia-alzheimer.html. Accessed September 10, 2014.

even stronger steroids, a bronchodilator and a nebulizer. What the pediatricians didn't tell me as well is that eczema and asthma are caused by the very same things that cause Sensory Processing Disorder: toxicity, gut dysbiosis, nutritional deficiencies, inflammation and hormonal imbalances. After learning about these causes and applying what I'm teaching you in this book, my son no longer has asthma or eczema.

Radiation

The only place I've ever seen radiation discussed in the context of neurodevelopmental disorders is in Laura Lambert Hirsch's *The Other Side of Autism*. Given the cumulative impacts of nuclear-bomb detonation, atomic bomb testing, Chernobyl and the two TRILLION becquerels of strontium-90 and cesium-137 that have leaked so far from the Fukushima power plant in Japan[52] – which is still leaking, by the way – it's just common sense that this level of radiation would have some detrimental effect on our health.

Radiation toxicity came up as the number one problem for both me and my older son when we were tested by Michelle Giliberto, a co-founder of Epidemic Answers who is also a vibrational remedy practitioner. It had to be dealt with before any other health issues could. Sadly, I'm not surprised, given that I grew up four miles down the road from the Oak Ridge National Lab's (ORNL) K-25 uranium enrichment plant in Oak Ridge, TN, where the first atomic bomb was built. The plant is still in operation, and *The Fluoride Deception* describes how low-level radioactive waste in the form of uranyl fluroide was at toxic levels in the area for decades.[53] I believe it must have gotten into the groundwater that my family drank and bathed in on a daily basis. No wonder my mother's health

---

52. http://www.japantimes.co.jp/news/2014/09/07/national/two-trillion-becquerels-radioactive-material-may-escaped-1/#.VBC2Qkh8HYv. Accessed September 10, 2014.
53. Bryson, C. *The Fluoride Deception*. New York, NY: Seven Stories Press, 2004, 279.

declined so rapidly when we moved to the area and she began work as an information analyst at ORNL. In any case, as with all of these causes that I am discussing, it must have been passed on from me to my son when I was pregnant with him.

Endocrine Disruptors

When you see the term "endocrine disruptor," think "thyroid and adrenal damager," so not only do endocrine disruptors damage the thyroid and adrenals, but they also damage the reproductive system and its hormones, which may, in my mind, be one of the real reasons for the rise in neurodevelopmental disorders, infertility and the reduction in age of puberty.

There is no end to the tricks that endocrine disruptors can play on our bodies: increasing production of certain hormones; decreasing production of others; imitating hormones; turning one hormone into another; interfering with hormone signaling; telling cells to die prematurely; competing with essential nutrients; binding to essential hormones; accumulating in organs that produce hormones.

Pesticides

Pesticides damage your child's nervous and endrocrine systems.[54] After all, that's how they were designed to kill those pests. Pesticides and other toxins in food are linked to cancer, developmental delays and birth defects. Eating organic food would avoid these risks.[55]

Even low levels of and prenatal exposure to organophosphate pesticides cause neurodevelopmental

---

54. Korrick, S., et al, Polychlorinated Biphenyls (PCBs), Organochlorine Pesticides, and Neurodevelopment, *Curr Opin Pediatr.* Apr 2008; 20(2): 10.1097/MOP.0b013e3282f6a4e9.

55. Vogt, Rainbow, et al, Cancer and non-cancer health effects from food contaminant exposures for children and adults in California: a risk assessment, *Environmental Health* 2012, 11:83 .

damage.[56] Exposure is linked to a decline in memory and slower processing speed.[57] Organophosphate pesticides have been linked to ADHD, concluded the authors of a study in *Pediatrics*: "Each 10-fold increase in urinary concentration of organophosphate metabolites was associated with a 55 percent to 72 percent increase in the odds of ADHD."[58]

Organochlorine pesticides may decrease T3 thyroid hormone during early life, leading to hypothyroidism and damaging a child's neurodevelopment.[59]

The pesticide Roundup® (glyphosate) significantly increases the bioaccumulation of mercury.[60] In addition, researchers now believe that it might not be gluten that's the problem in people with celiac disease and gluten intolerance; instead, the use of Roundup® on wheat may actually be causing these issues.[61] Dietrich Klinghardt, MD, PhD believes that Roundup® is the number one reason for thyroid dysfunction.

It might not be the food itself that's causing the health issue; it might be what's been done to it as was found with the use of pesticides known as dichlorophenols, such as the pesticide 2,4-D.[62] In fact, Vani Hari, aka Food Babe, has said

---

56. Shelton, J.F., et al, Neurodevelopmental Disorders and Prenatal Residential Proximity to Agricultural Pesticides: The CHARGE Study, *Environ Health Perspect.* 2014 Jun 23. [Epub ahead of print]
57. Ross, Sarah Mackenzie, et al, Neurobehavioral problems following low-level exposure to organophosphate pesticides: a systematic and meta-analytic review, *Critical Reviews in Toxicology*, 2012; 1.
58. Bouchard, Maryse F., PhD, et al, Attention-Deficit/Hyperactivity Disorder and Urinary Metabolites of Organophosphate Pesticides, *Pediatrics.* Jun 2010; 125(6): e1270–e1277.
59. Mnif, W., et al, Effect of endocrine disruptor pesticides: a review, *Int J Environ Res Public Health.* 2011 Jun;8(6):2265-303.
60. Tsui, M.T., et al, Influence of glyphosate and its formulation (Roundup) on the toxicity and bioavailability of metals to Ceriodaphnia dubia, *Environ Pollut.* 2005 Nov;138(1):59-68.
61. Samsel, A. and Seneff, S. Glyphosate, pathways to modern diseases II: Celiac sprue and gluten intolerance, *Interdiscip Toxicol.* Dec 2013; 6(4): 159–184.
62. Jerschow, E., et al, Dichlorophenol-containing pesticides and allergies results from the US National Health and Nutrition Examination Survey

that she thought she was allergic to spinach when she was younger, but she later discovered that when she ate organic spinach, she didn't have a reaction; the pesticides were the problem.[63] Dichlorophenols are also found in moth balls and room deodorizers. Because they kill bacteria, including the good bacteria in your child's gut, they may thus contribute to gut dysbiosis.

Phthalates

These chemicals are one of the most insidious because they are everywhere in most, if not all, plastics and in many personal-care products. They're also in food and beverage packaging and leach into food. Phthalates give plastics that "rubber ducky" feel and are often found in children's toys. They're oh so cute, but oh so toxic, as 75% of children's Disney, Spider-Man and Dora the Explorer back-to-school products had high levels of phthalates.[64] I can't confirm it, but I personally believe that many pens with special grips and OXO Good Grips kitchen tools contain high levels of phthalates.

Dr. Sherry Rogers, author of *Detoxify or Die*, says that they are the number one toxin in our lives[65], as over 97% of people tested positive for phthalate exposure.[66] In addition, they are highly linked to diabetes.[67] Prenatal exposure to phthalates has

---

2005-2006, *Ann Allergy Asthma Immunol.* 2012 Dec;109(6):420-5.

63. https://www.facebook.com/thefoodbabe/posts/834417106593002. Accessed September 11, 2014.

64. http://chej.org/2012/08/hiddenhazardsrelease/. Accessed September 11, 2014.

65. Rogers, Sherry A., MD, *Detoxify or Die.* Sarasota, FL: Sand Key Company, Inc., 2002, 2.

66. Teitelbaum SL, Associations between phthalate metabolite urinary concentrations and body size measures in New York City children, *Environ Res.* 2012 Jan;112:186-93.

67. James-Todd, T., Urinary phthalate metabolite concentrations and diabetes among women in the National Health and Nutrition Examination Survey (NHANES) 2001-2008, *Environ Health Perspect.* 2012 Sep;120(9):1307-13.

been linked to lower mental and gross motor scores in infants, particularly boys.[68]

BPA and BPS

BPA is typically found in canned foods and polycarbonate plastics, but because something is labeled "BPA free" doesn't mean it's safe. In fact, it usually contains a more harmful, less known bisphenol: BPS. Both of these are potent, yet pervasive, endocrine disruptors that have been found to cause neurodevelopmental damage.[69]

Fluoride

Fluoride is commonly found in fluoridated toothpaste, drinking water, and anti-depressants, yet it suppresses the thyroid by displacing iodine. Thyroid suppressers affect a child's neurodevelopment. In a meta-analysis of the effects of fluoride on children's neurodevelopment, researchers concluded that, "The results support the possibility of an adverse effect of high fluoride exposure on children's neurodevelopment."[70]

We've been sold a pile of crap in thinking that fluoride is necessary for our dental health; it's not. Fluoride is a byproduct of uranium enrichment, and Edward Bernays – the "Father of Spin" – was the man who figured out how to take a toxic byproduct and make everyone believe that it's good for them. On Wall Street, this is known as "putting lipstick on a pig." I highly suggest you read *The Fluoride Deception* by Bryan

---

68. Kim, Y., et al, Prenatal exposure to phthalates and infant development at six months: Prospective Mothers and Children's Environmental Health (MOCEH) Study, *Environ Health Perspect.* 2011 Oct;119(10):1495-500.
69. Kaur, K., Bisphenol A induces oxidative stress and mitochondrial dysfunction in lymphoblasts from children with autism and unaffected siblings, *Free Radic Biol* Med. 2014 Aug 4;76C:25-33.
70. Choi, A.L., et al, Developmental fluoride neurotoxicity: a systematic review and meta-analysis, *Environ Health Perspect.* 2012 Oct;120(10):1362-8.

Christenson to understand the history of how we've been duped in this mass con.

Chlorine

Chlorine is another halide chemical, as are fluoride, bromine and iodine. These elements have the same electron valence, meaning that they easily displace each other. Thus, chlorine kicks out necessary iodine in your child's body. Chlorine is commonly found in drinking and swimming-pool water, pesticides and Splenda®, and it's been linked to a rising number of people with food allergies, most likely because it is an endocrine disruptor that also kills good gut flora.[71]

Flame Retardants

Brominated flame retardants (PBDE) are neurotoxic and are linked to neurodevelopmental disorders such as Sensory Processing Disorder, autism and ADHD. Researchers found that "PBDE exposure was associated with changes in the motor function and the serum levels of the thyroid hormones."[72] Flame retardants are pervasive, as they are found in children's sleepwear, Mountain Dew, fabric furniture, mattresses and electrical/computer-cable coverings.[73] The newer the furniture is the more flame retardants it has.

---

71. Jerschow, E., et al, Dichlorophenol-containing pesticides and allergies results from the US National Health and Nutrition Examination Survey 2005-2006, *Ann Allergy Asthma Immunol.* 2012 Dec;109(6):420-5.

72. Kiciński M[1], et al, Neurobehavioral function and low-level exposure to brominated flame retardants in adolescents: a cross-sectional study, *Environ Health.* 2012 Nov 14;11:86.

73. http://well.blogs.nytimes.com/2014/07/01/flame-retardants-are-everywhere. Accessed September 11, 2014.

Teflon®

Teflon® and other non-stick coatings like water-proofing chemicals belong to a group of chemicals known as perfluorinated compounds (PFCs). The most common ones are perfluoro-octane sulphonate (PFOS) and perfluorooctanoic acid (PFOA). Not only do these chemicals disrupt the endocrine system, but they are also neurotoxic and can create an autoimmune response. Researchers discovered that "developmental exposure to PFOA may induce immunotoxicity similar to that observed in subsets of patients with neurodevelopmental disorders" because it affects the immune system's T cell responses.[74]

Parabens

These environmental toxins are also found in many personal-care products such as soaps, shampoos, lotions as well as cough syrups because they prevent bacteria growth. They are usually in the form of ethylparaben, methylparaben, propylparaben and butylparaben. Not only are they endocrine disruptors, but they can cause neurodevelopmental damage. Researchers found that "prenatal exposure to butyl paraben induced neuro-developmental disorders similar to some of the neurodevelopmental disorders observed in the VA model of autism."[75]

---

74. Hu, Q., et al, Does developmental exposure to perflurooctanoic acid (PFOA) induce immunopathologies commonly observed in neurodevelopmental disorders?, *Neurotoxicology*. 2012 Dec;33(6):1491-8.
75. Ali, E.H., et al, Combined prenatal and postnatal butyl paraben exposure produces autism-like symptoms in offspring: comparison with valproic acid autistic model, *Pharmacol Biochem Behav*. 2013 Oct;111:102-10.

Triclosan

Not only is triclosan, the drug in many anti-bacterial hand sanitizers and soaps, an endocrine disruptor (it damages your child's thyroid gland, adrenal glands and hormonal system) and a pesticide (it kills your child's good gut flora), but now researchers are finding out it leads to muscle weakness – including cardiac weakness – Parkinson's, multiple sclerosis and heart disease. In addition, use of triclosan is associated with allergies: "Triclosan levels measured in urine were associated with elevated levels of Immunoglobulin E (IgE) and rhinitis (blocked nose/hay fever) in 10 year-olds."[76] Triclosan has also been linked to cancer-cell growth.[77]

Goitrogenic Foods

Raw cruciferous vegetables and some other foods can disrupt the function of the thyroid. Foods such as broccoli, cauliflower, bok choy, cabbage, Brussels sprouts, kale, collard greens and spinach are goitrogenic when raw, although it takes cooking them for about an hour and a half to fully destroy goitrogens. The Weston A. Price Foundation says that a "small amount of goitrogens ... is not harmful if one's diet is adequate in iodine."[78]

Unfermented Soy

Unfermented soy in the form of tofu, soy milk, soy

---

76. Bertelsen, R.J., Triclosan exposure and allergic sensitization in Norwegian children, *Allergy*. 2013 Jan;68(1):84-91.
77. Lee, Hye-Rim, et al, Progression of Breast Cancer Cells Was Enhanced by Endocrine-Disrupting Chemicals, Triclosan and Octylphenol, via an Estrogen Receptor-Dependent Signaling Pathway in Cellular and Mouse Xenograft Models, *Chem. Res. Toxicol.*, 2014, 27 (5), pp 834–842.
78. http://www.westonaprice.org/health-topics/abcs-of-nutrition/bearers-of-the-cross-crucifers-in-the-context-of-traditional-diets-and-modern-science/#goitrogens. Accessed September 11, 2014.

formula, soy protein isolates (found in most protein bars), edamame and other raw forms of soy can also disrupt the thyroid because these are goitrogenic foods.[79] The amount of processing that it takes to extract soy protein and tofu is mind-blowing. It's not real food if it's gone through this much processing. In addition, The Cornucopia Institute revealed the dirty little secret of processed soy in its report, "Behind the Bean: The Heroes and Charlatans of the Natural and Organic Soy Foods Industry," which is that hexane is widely used in the processing of soy. Hexane is a neurotoxic petrochemical that is prohibited in the production of organic foods, but "is used to make "natural" soy foods and even some that are "made with organic ingredients," such as Clif Bars®."[80]

Just because a food is marketed as healthy doesn't mean that it is. In fact, I recommend you avoid giving your child any kind of food that's making a health claim because I've found that these processed, junk foods are using the claim to divert you from the fact that they're not healthy. Do you see fresh produce listed with a health claim?

Mold

Ritchie Shoemaker, MD of www.survivingmold.com estimates that roughly half of American households have some form of mold toxicity. Mold can lurk undetected in heating and cooling systems, as well as behind walls and in the basement. Mycotoxins from mold dispersed into the air from these organisms can cause runny noses, itchy eyes, coughing, headaches, breathing difficulties, achiness, multiple sclerosis, fibromyalgia, fatigue and problems with the executive function of the brain including memory and concentration.

Personally, I've known quite a few children with Sensory Processing Disorder, autism and ADHD whose parents

79. http://www.westonaprice.org/health-topics/the-ploy-of-soy/. Accessed September 11, 2014.
80. http://www.cornucopia.org/2009/05/soy-report-and-scorecard/#more-1375. Accessed September 11, 2014.

discovered that there was a horrible mold problem in the house, sometimes hidden inside the walls. Just because you can't see it doesn't mean it's not there. I highly recommend you read *My House Is Killing Me! The Home Guide for Families with Allergies and Asthma* by Jeffrey C. May as well as *Is This Your Child?* by Doris Rapp, MD to learn more about this more-common-than-we-think problem.

EMFs

Chronic exposure to electromagnetic fields puts your child's body in a state of stress, even when resting. Research shows EMF can cause changes in both the sympathetic nervous system as well as the parasympathetic nervous system, and researchers described the top 10 symptoms of EMF sensitivity as:

- Memory problems
- Difficulty concentrating
- Eye problems
- Sleep problems
- Feeling unwell
- Headache
- Dizziness
- Tinnitus
- Chronic fatigue
- Heart palpitations[81]

Common sources of EMF exposure are fluorescent lights, cell phones, cordless house phones, baby monitors, Wi-Fi systems, smart meters and large electric devices such as refrigerators. My top two sources for understanding this issue in more detail

81.http://www.researchgate.net/publication/228993615_Provocation_study_using_heart_rate_variability_shows_microwave_radiation_from_2.4_GHz_cordless_phone_affects_autonomic_nervous_system. Accessed September 11, 2014.

are Ann Louise Gittleman's book *Zapped: Why Your Cell Phone Shouldn't Be Your Alarm Clock and 1,268 Ways to Outsmart the Hazards of Electronic Pollution* and the Electric Sense website, www.electricsense.com.

Perfumes and Scented Products

Synthetic fragrances, colognes and perfumes are typically made from petrochemicals, and researchers have discovered that they can cause acute toxic effects.[82] The Environmental Working Group's Skin Deep cosmetic database lists some of the toxic effects of fragrance as:

- Ecotoxicology
- Allergies/immunotoxicity
- Irritation (skin, eyes, or lungs)
- Organ system toxicity (non-reproductive)

In addition, preservatives and additives such as BHT, butylphenyl methylpropional, hydroxycitronellal, geraniol, cinnamyl alcohol, isoeugenol, limonene and others that are typically used in these products can cause:

- Biochemical or cellular level changes
- Endocrine disruption
- Persistence and bioaccumulation
- Cancer

Synthetic fragrances can trigger rashes, eczema, allergies and asthma. They add to the toxic burden of an already toxic body, and many SPD kids are extremely sensitive to them, even in the form of scented soaps, laundry detergent and dryer sheets. This kind of chemical sensitivity is indicative of a congested liver.

---

82. Anderson, R.C., Acute toxic effects of fragrance products, *Arch Environ Health.* 1998 Mar-Apr;53(2):138-46.

Carcinogens

You would think that in this day and age with all of the government agencies in existence that are supposedly guarding our health and well-being that carcinogens would not be a part of our children's daily lives, but they are.

Formaldehyde and Dioxane

Formaldehyde is a known carcinogen that's used for embalming dead bodies, and the EPA has classified 1,4-dioxane as a possible carcinogen Believe it or not, these are ingredients in some personal-care products, such as Johnson & Johnson's BABY products. For decades, Americans have come to believe that Johnson & Johnson's products are perhaps the best choice for their babies. I know that when my boys were little, I was given lots of little samples of their shampoos, body washes and powders for babies.

Now, Johnson & Johnson is finally yielding to pressure and changing the formulas of their personal-care products to remove known carcinogens: formaldehyde (released by the ubiquitous quaternium-15) and 1,4-dioxane. WHY WERE THESE ALLOWED TO BE IN THERE IN THE FIRST PLACE?

I think it's because we've collectively fallen asleep at the wheel. I think most Americans assume, as I used to, that if it's sold in a store, it must be safe because surely the FDA has tested it for safety. NOT TRUE. The sad thing is that we've placed our trust in this and other companies because we've been led to believe, by millions of dollars spent on marketing and advertising, that their products are safe.

Another example of formaldehyde hidden in plain sight is that it is a product of the breakdown of the artificial sweetener aspartame, brought to you by Monsanto, of course. Aspartame has been linked to seizures, multiple sclerosis, fibromyalgia, migraines[83] and more. No wonder! Aspartame is the sweetener of choice in diet drinks and sugar-free "foods" and candies.

Styrene

Styrene (vinylbenzene) is listed as "reasonably anticipated to be a human carcinogen" and is used to make plastics, rubber and resins. Polystyrene is Styrofoam, and the chemical leaches out of Styrofoam food containers and cups when something hot is in it. I am amazed that restaurants are still allowed to sell food and drinks in Styrofoam containers.

Dioxin

Dioxins are a group of hundreds of chemicals that are highly persistent in the environment, and the most toxic one of them is 2,3,7,8-tetrachlorodibenzo-p-dioxin or TCDD, a known carcinogen.[84] A draft report by the EPA in 1994 stated that there is no safe level exposure to dioxin, yet it is still found in diapers, tampons and sanitary pads as a bleaching agent.

Agent Orange, an herbicide used in the Vietnam War, is a 50/50 blend of 2,4-D and 2,4,5-T, and dioxin is a byproduct of 2,4,5-T. Veterans of the war who came in contact with Agent Orange have significantly higher rates of cancer. Dow Agroscience continues to manufacture 2,4-D and uses it in Scott's Weed and Feed, Miracle-Grow Weed and Feed, Weed B Gone.[85]

This issue has personal meaning to me because my dad was an organic chemist in Dow's Midland, MI, facility in the 1950s and 1960s. He held patents for the development of 2, 4, 6, 8-tetra-tertiarybutylphenoxazine, 2-halo-4, 6-ditertiaryalkyl

---

83. Jacob, S.E., Formaldehyde, aspartame, and migraines: a possible connection, *Dermatitis*, 2008 May-Jun;19(3):E10-1.
84. http://www.ejnet.org/dioxin/. Accessed September 13, 2014.
85. http://www.agentorangerecord.com/information/what_is_dioxin/. Accessed September 13, 2014.

phenol esters, halo-dicyclohexyl-phenols, halogenated coal acids, polyurethane and various coal-acid applications, many of which were used to make pesticides. The Midland plant produced chlorpyrifos, pentachlorphenol, 2,4-D and 2,4,5-T, dioxins, styrene, benzene, vinyl chloride and arsenic, and has a documented significantly higher cancer rate among its employees.[86] My dad died at the young age of 57 from a rare combination of bone-marrow and stomach cancers; this combination was found only in his unit at the Midland facility. Although my mom didn't work there, it's possible that he exposed her to these chemicals, as many chemical workers are known to "carry" them home, especially back in those days when people didn't understand the toxicity of the chemicals they were surrounded by.

Carrageenan

Carrageenan is a potential carcinogen made by processing red seaweed. It's used as a thickener in ice cream, soups non-dairy milks, and even in organic versions of these "foods." It's also found in deli meats and low-fat foods. Carrageenan has been linked to gastrointestinal inflammation. A review of the scientific literature was performed in 2001 stating that "because of the acknowledged carcinogenic properties of degraded carrageenan in animal models and the cancer-promoting effects of undegraded carrageenan in experimental models, the widespread use of carrageenan in the Western diet should be reconsidered," yet the additive continues to show up in "foods."[87]

86. Burns, C.J., Cause-specific mortality among Michigan employees of a chemical company: 1940 to 1994, *J Occup Environ Med.* 2002 Feb;44(2):168-75.
87. Tobacman, J.K., Review of harmful gastrointestinal effects of carrageenan in animal experiments, *Environ Health Perspect.* Oct 2001; 109(10): 983–994.

Polycyclic Aromatic Hydrocarbons

Toluene, benzene and xylene are petrochemicals known as polycyclic aromatic hydrocarbons, and they are a component of car exhaust. Toluene is also a component of some nail polishes that also typically contain phthalates and formaldehyde. While benzene is a known carcinogen, xylene and toluene are not classified as such. However, research indicates that "there is recent evidence of carcinogenicity of toluene and xylene at high concentrations in experimental animals."[88] A team of researchers concluded that "exposure to traffic-related air pollution…during pregnancy and during the first year of life was associated with autism."[89]

Vinyl

Vinyl chloride, usually known as just "vinyl," is a known carcinogen. It's found in PVC pipes, shower curtains, flooring material, children's toys, wire and cable coatings, and packaging materials, and has been linked as a potential cause of autism.[90]

PCBs

Polychlorinated biphenyls, otherwise known as PCBs, are a group of persistent organic pollutants that are known carcinogens. Although they are no longer made or used in the United States, they are still found in power transformers, soil and water, as well as in breast milk. "There is growing evidence to support an association between PCBs and deficits

---

88. McMichael, A.J., Carcinogenicity of benzene, toluene and xylene: epidemiological and experimental evidence, *IARC Sci Publ.* 1988;(85):3-18.
89. Volk, H.E., Traffic-related air pollution, particulate matter, and autism, *JAMA Psychiatry.* 2013 Jan;70(1):71-7.
90. Larsson, M., et al, Associations between indoor environmental factors and parental-reported autistic spectrum disorders in children 6-8 years of age, *Neurotoxicology.* 2009 Sep;30(5):822-31.

of neurodevelopment" says a team of researchers,[91] and PCBs have been shown to cause symptoms of ADHD.[92]

Standard American Diet (SAD)

The Standard American Diet isn't what it used to be. Your grandmother wouldn't recognize what we call "food" as food because, many times, it's not. With the advent of GMOs (genetically modified organisms), artificial colors, artificial flavors, "natural" flavors, flavor enhancers, artificial sweeteners, preservatives and other food additives to processed foods – which is what most people eat these days, the food that our children eat is downright toxic.

I, too, used to trust the FDA and USDA, thinking that if it's sold in a store, it must be safe. Those were carefree days. These days, I've had to become a food vigilante to protect the health of myself and my children because as Ann Wigmore said, "The food you eat can be either the safest and most powerful form of medicine or the slowest form of poison."

GMOs

GMO foods are foods that have been genetically modified, and very little safety testing has been done on them. The proteins in these foods have been genetically modified and are foreign to the human body, causing an allergy or sensitivity to them. There have been no human clinical trials testing their safety. Instead, the FDA relies on GMO companies, such as Monsanto to self-police, most likely because Michael Taylor, a

---

91. Park, H.Y., et al, Neurodevelopmental toxicity of prenatal polychlorinated biphenyls (PCBs) by chemical structure and activity: a birth cohort study, *Environ Health.* 2010 Aug 23;9:51.
92. Sazonova, N.A., et al, Transcriptome-wide gene expression in a rat model of attention deficit hyperactivity disorder symptoms: rats developmentally exposed to polychlorinated biphenyls, *Am J Med Genet B Neuropsychiatr Genet.* 2011 Dec;156B(8):898-912.

former Vice President and lobbyist for Monsanto, was the FDA's Food Safety Czar when GMOs were allowed into the food supply without being tested. As another example of a conflict of interest, Supreme Court Justice Clarence Thomas, who once worked for Monsanto as a lawyer, wrote the majority opinion on a decision involving Monsanto's plant patents. These are just two high-profile examples; to learn more about food-industry manipulation and political collusion, I urge you to read *Seeds of Deception: Exposing Industry and Government Lies About the Safety of the Genetically Engineered Foods You're Eating* by Jeffrey Smith, the head of the Institute for Responsible Technology.

Robyn O'Brien's book, *The Unhealthy Truth: One Mother's Shocking Investigation into the Dangers of America's Food Supply – and What Every Family Can Do to Protect Itself*, is a shocking investigation into the many ways we've been tricked into eating not just unhealthy, but downright dangerous, food., especially GMO foods. Robyn discovered that many of the peer-reviewed research studies about allergies are funded by industry, especially Monsanto. So all of this blind faith that we've had in "science" is shattered after we realize that the "science" can be made to say whatever industry wants it to. Robyn advises us to research the funding source of an expert opinion by Googling the name of the doctor with terms like "funding," "consulting fee," "grant," or "disclosure".[93] Unfortunately, these days, you have to learn to think for yourself and assume that the source of the payment may have a negative effect on the expert's ability to be impartial and unbiased.

Throughout her book, Robyn, with the thoroughness of the Wall Street analyst that she used to be, details her investigations of how she discovered that the foxes are guarding the hen house and how Big Ag and Big Pharma are in bed with the government that we thought was protecting us so that people become long-term profit centers. There's a

---

93. O'Brien, Robyn, *The Unhealthy Truth: One Mother's Shocking Investigation into the Dangers of America's Food Supply – and What Every Family Can Do to Protect Itself.* New York, NY: Broadway Books, 2009, 196.

(somewhat) famous saying, at least in my world these days, from Wendell Berry that says, "People are fed by the food industry, which pays no attention to health, and treated by the health industry, which pays no attention to food." I would say this quote captures the essence of Robyn's book.

In any case, the reason Robyn was led to her investigations is the same reason I was led to mine: something was wrong with the health of her children. One day after eating breakfast, her daughter's face grew so red and puffy that her eyes couldn't open. It led Robyn down a path that many of us these days have had to go down: questioning authority, including our pediatricians, FDA and USDA, people and agencies that we were taught to trust.

She discovered that the very organization that many of us thought was out there to help us with our children's food allergies, FAAN (Food Allergy & Anapyhlaxis Network) – now calling itself FARE (Food Allergy Research & Education) – is nothing but a shill, a fake non-profit front solely owned by Kraft. Robyn discovered this sickening fact after doing her due diligence and after being told to "cease and desist" by them – you'll have to read the book for the whole story.

Robyn compellingly shows us in this book that many of these authorities can't be trusted. She exposes Monsanto for the fraud that they are and points out how their genetically modified (GMO) foods – soy and corn – as well as their bovine-growth formula (rBGH) that's in non-organic dairy these days are linked to the staggering increases in allergies, asthma, ADHD and cancer. Jeffrey Smith's book, *Genetic Roulette: The Documented Health Risks of Genetically Modified Foods*, as well as his non-profit Institute for Responsible Technology reveal that GMO foods have been linked to:

- Allergies
- Asthma
- ADHD
- Cancer
- Gluten disorders

- Autism
- Liver problems
- Infant mortality
- Reproductive problems
- Sterility

GMO foods have either been engineered to release pesticides upon consumption, as in the case of Bt corn, which roughly 95% of non-organic corn is these days, or they've been engineered to withstand very high doses of the toxic pesticide Roundup®, otherwise known as glyphosate. In fact, Stephanie Seneff, PhD, has documented that the real reason that there are so many more people with gluten intolerance and celiac disease these days is due to the Roundup® that's sprayed on food crops such as wheat, soybeans and corn.[94] That's why they're called "Roundup® ready" crops.

Consider the fact that GMOs are illegal in Europe and most of the rest of the world, even China and Russia. Also consider the fact that the Grocery Manufacturers Association has spent millions of dollars ($47 million in California in 2012 alone)[95] to sway public opinion and to keep voters from voting to have GMOs labeled. What are they hiding? These are the big Big Food companies such as Monsanto, Kraft, Coca-Cola, Pepsi, Campbell Soups, Nestlé and Dupont. They have spent millions to defeat GMO-labeling laws in other states, too, like Washington, Maine and Connecticut.

I recommend that your child avoid eating all non-organic versions of soy, corn, sugar beets and canola, as there's a 95% chance that they are genetically modified; by law, organic foods cannot be genetically modified. I also recommend that your child not eat organic versions either because unfermented soy is an endocrine disruptor, corn is full of inflammatory omega-

---

94. Samsel, A. and Seneff, S. Glyphosate, pathways to modern diseases II: Celiac sprue and gluten intolerance, *Interdiscip Toxicol.* Dec 2013; 6(4): 159–184.

95. http://www.cornucopia.org/2014/06/grocery-manufacturers-fail-squelch-money-laundering-lawsuit/. Accessed September 4, 2014.

6's, and canola oil is an inflammatory vegetable oil. When you buy processed food or eat out in a restaurant, though, it's hard to avoid these foods. Restaurants and food companies prefer them because they are cheap.

Artificial Colors

Artificial colors are those "FD&C" colors that you see on the label of processed foods, and they're in most children's foods these days, as well as cough syrups, decongestants, mouthwashes and toothpastes. They have never been tested for safety, and they are highly linked to behavioral problems in children. Artificial colors are made from petroleum and can contain carcinogens such as benzidine and heavy metals like lead.[96] The Feingold Association of the United States has thoroughly documented with peer-reviewed medical research the negative health effects of artificial colors, which have been linked to:

- ADD/ADHD
- Allergies
- Asthma
- Autism/PDD-NOS/Asperger's
- Autoimmune conditions
- Bedwetting
- Behavioral disorders
- Depression
- Earaches
- Eczema
- GI problems
- Headaches
- Learning problems
- Seizures
- Sleep problems

As an example, Kraft puts the artificial color tartrazine in

96. http://feingold.org/6certified.php. Accessed September 4, 2014.

their macaroni and cheese; I used to willingly give this to my kids. Tartrazine, for those of you who don't know, is a petroleum-derived artificial color that is linked to hyperactivity in children and, in America, is listed on the label as FD&C #5. The telling and sad point is that the macaroni and other foods that Kraft sells in Europe don't contain tartrazine because of the prudence of the European Union. It's a telling point because it tells you how deep the corruption runs over here in the states.

Artificial Flavors

Beware of any food product that lists artificial flavors on its label. You really have no idea what's in there, although you can know for sure that it is a mix of chemicals, not food, that is derived from artificial sources. For example, did you know that artificial butter flavoring can cause long-term neurological toxicity?[97]

You assume that the orange juice you buy in the store is safe, right? Did you know it's been likely sitting in vats for at least a year after having its flavor stripped out and then had artificial flavors and ethyl butyrate, a petrochemical with a pineapple flavor that's also used in perfumes, added back in? These ingredients aren't listed on the label, and you can read more about this scandal in *Squeezed: What You Don't Know About Orange Juice* by Alissa Hamilton. In the meantime, if you want to give your family orange juice, I recommend squeezing it yourself!

Natural Flavors

Ingredients listed on the label as "natural flavors" may not be any better for your child than artificial flavors. The truth is we just don't know what's in those flavors except that they

97. More, S.S., et al, The butter flavorant, diacetyl, exacerbates β-amyloid cytotoxicity, *Chem Res Toxicol.* 2012 Oct 15;25(10):2083-91.

were originally sourced from a natural product; remember, though, that "natural" is a meaningless term, as it's not backed up by any certification process. Most times, natural flavors are made in laboratories, too. For example, sometimes vanilla flavoring is actually from beaver anal gland secretions, which technically is natural, but I'm sure that's not what you thought your child was eating!

Flavor Enhancers

Flavor enhancers are chemicals that have been specifically designed to trick you into thinking that something tastes sweeter, saltier or more savory. Monsodium glutamate is the most well known flavor enhancer, as I discuss in "Other Food Sensitivities," Be sure to avoid food products with labels that have MSG, autolyzed yeast, hydrolyzed, textured vegetable protein or other MSG aliases listed.

Flavor enhancers allow food manufacturers to say "low sugar", "low fat" or "no MSG" on the label. The problem is that flavor enhancers are not always listed in a food product's ingredients label. The really disgusting thing is that Senomyx, a large flavor enhancer manufacturing company that sells its enhancers to food manufacturers such as Kraft, Pepsi and Nestlé, makes some of these flavor enhancers from the tissue of aborted human fetuses.[98] I'm not kidding. *Now* will you stop feeding your child processed foods?

Artificial Sweeteners

Although saccharin, which was commonly used as a sugar replacement for diabetics, was listed as a carcinogen in 1981 because of the fear that it potentially causes cancer,[99] it was delisted in 2000. My thought is that if a food product comes

---

98. http://articles.mercola.com/sites/articles/archive/2013/03/17/senomyx-flavor-enhancers.aspx. Accessed September 5, 2014.

99. Reuber, M.D., Carcinogenicity of saccharin, *Environ Health Perspect.* Aug 1978; 25: 173–200.

directly from a plant or animal, then it's fine to eat as long as it's not poisonous; if it's not, then don't. As Michael Pollan wrote in *Food Rules*, "If it comes from a plant, eat it. If it was made in a plant, don't."

- **Aspartame** usually shows up on the label of diet soft drinks and sugar-free foods these days. It goes under the brand names NutraSweet® and Equal®. Aspartame-sweetened sodas exposed to higher temperatures turn into poisonous wood alcohol (methanol). Methanol turns into carcinogenic formaldehyde,[100] which can cause migraines, allergies, seizures, as well as symptoms of lupus, Parkinson's, Alzheimer's, autism, multiple sclerosis and fibromyalgia.[101] One of my nieces has epilepsy, and she stopped having seizures after she stopped drinking diet sodas.
- **Neotame** is the newest artificial sweetener and a derivative of aspartame. It has been found to cause headaches, liver toxicity and low birth rate.[102]
- **Splenda®** (sucralose) can cause diarrhea, migraines and thymus shrinkage;[103] the thymus is a critical gland for immune function, especially in newborns and children. Splenda® contributes to gut dysbiosis, as it was found to cut beneficial gut flora IN HALF while also increasing acidity.[104] Chemically, Splenda® is similar to DDT, as it is a highly chlorinated molecule. Although Splenda® has also been found to cause migraines, seizures, dizziness GI problems and dizziness,[105] it is often added to

---

100. Jacob, S.E., Formaldehyde, aspartame, and migraines: a possible connection, *Dermatitis*. 2008 May-Jun;19(3):E10-1.
101. Whitehouse, C.R., et al, The potential toxicity of artificial sweeteners, *AAOHN J*. 2008 Jun;56(6):251-9; quiz 260-1.
102. Ibid, 256.
103. Ibid.
104. Abou-Donia M.B., et al, Splenda alters gut microflora and increases intestinal p-glycoprotein and cytochrome p-450 in male rats, *J Toxicol Environ Health A*. 2008;71(21):1415-29.
105. http://articles.mercola.com/sites/articles/archive/2009/02/10/new-study-of-splenda-reveals-shocking-information-about-potential-harmful-

pharmaceuticals without being listed on the label. Splenda® also releases carcinogenic dioxin when it's heated.[106]

In February 2013, the dairy industry petitioned the FDA to add aspartame, sucralose and/or other artificial sweeteners to milk and dairy products *without the identification of those sweeteners on the label.* Let's hope that petition doesn't get granted, but I am thoroughly disgusted that an industry would be so deceitful as to intentionally hide these health-damaging substances in our foods without our knowledge.

Preservatives

Almost by definition, processed foods need preservatives to keep them from turning moldy or going bad. Preservatives are the reason that your McDonald's food or other fast food, junk food or processed food looks the same now as it will in a year if you leave it out, unrefrigerated. The problem is that these preservatives are usually damaging to our health. The most common ones are:

- **Sodium benzoate** is a mold inhibitor commonly found in processed foods such as soft drinks, pickles and sauces. It turns into benzene, a known carcinogen, when mixed with vitamins C and E.[107] Remember that mercury is used to produce sodium benzoate.
- **Sodium nitrite** is often found in processed meats like bacon, ham, hot dogs, corned beef, luncheon meats and smoked fish. The consumption of it is linked with various types of cancer, such as pancreatic cancer.[108]

---

effects.aspx. Accessed September 5, 2014.

106. Schiffman, S.S., et al, Sucralose, a synthetic organochlorine sweetener: overview of biological issues. *J Toxicol Environ Health* B Crit Rev. 2013;16(7):399-451.

107. http://www.inchem.org/documents/cicads/cicads/cicad26.htm #SubSectionNumber:11.1.1. Accessed September 5, 2014.

108. Nöthlings U., et al, Meat and fat intake as risk factors for pancreatic

- **BHA and BHT** (butylated hydroxyanisole and butylated hydrozyttoluene) are potential carcinogens that are often found in cereals, potato chips and vegetable oils. These can cause symptoms ranging from mood swings, nausea, hives, asthma, headache and diarrhea to behavioral problems and sleeping problems.[109]
- **TBHQ** (tert-Butylhydroquinone), a petrochemical that is a form of lighter fluid, is found in chicken nuggets and other processed foods such as crackers. It can cause nausea, vomiting, collapse and ringing in the ears.[110]

Other Food Additives

As if there's not enough to worry about, there are other nasty ingredients lurking in the Standard American Diet. Some of the most common ones are:

- **Carrageenan** is a potential carcinogen used as a thickener in foods such as dairy alternatives, ice creams and soups. It has been linked to intestinal inflammation and colon cancer.[111]
- **Dimethylpolysiloxane** is an anti-foaming agent made of silicone used in cosmetics and other products like Silly Putty that is found in food such as chicken nuggets. This additive has not undergone any significant safety studies on human health.
- **Azodicarbonamide** is a chemical foaming agent also known as the "yoga mat" chemical. Although Vani Hari, aka the Food Babe, successfully petitioned to have it

---

cancer: the multiethnic cohort study, *J Natl Cancer Inst.* 2005 Oct 5;97(19):1458-65.

109. http://www.examiner.com/article/bht-the-harmful-food-additive-your-everyday-diet. Accessed September 5, 2014.

110. http://articles.mercola.com/sites/articles/archive/2010/11/08/do-you-have-any-idea-of-the-chemicals-used-in-fast-food-chicken.aspx. September 5, 2014.

111. http://www.cornucopia.org/carrageenan-2013/. Accessed September 5, 2014.

removed from Subway sandwich bread in 2014, the chemical remains in the food products of nearly 500 items, including 130 brands of bread, of brands such as Pillsbury, Sara Lee, Shoprite, Safeway, Smucker's, Fleischman's, Jimmy Dean, Kroger, Little Debbie, Tyson and Wonder.[112]

Testing for Toxicity

These days, there are more options for testing your child for exposure to the toxins I've just described. However, most pediatricians won't be aware of them, as they are likely not even aware of the role that environmental toxins play in the etiology of diseases and disorders. As one of our former pediatricians said, "You don't live in a toxic waste dump," showing that she didn't know about the subject. When I asked her for toxin testing, she blew it off with, "I don't like those 'holistic' labs," again showing her ignorance. It's up to you to stand up for your child's health and seek out a practitioner that can order tests to check for heavy metals as well as other kinds of toxins.

Testing for Heavy Metals

There are a variety of ways to test your child for heavy metals. My caveat in the interpretation of these results is that "normal" results aren't necessarily the same thing as optimal. For all of these tests, your child's levels will be measured versus a large population of people. As you've realized by now, everyone has some level of toxicity, so you need to understand that "normal" includes all of this pooled toxicity.

Hair Test

The heavy metal hair test is safe for children because it's

112. http://www.ewg.org/release/yoga-mat-chemical-found-nearly-500-foods. Accessed September 5, 2014.

non-invasive. It only involves cutting a certain amount of hair from as close to the scalp as possible and mailing it off to a lab.

Urine Test

A provoked urine test shows what is called the "body burden" of heavy metals because the chelating agents pull them out of tissues and organs. This involves taking a dose of chelating agents like DMSA and/or EDTA and measuring the amount of heavy metals that are excreted in the urine. Some people argue that results are invalid because a person will always have higher levels of heavy metals in the urine after taking a chelator. My rebuttal is that if the metals weren't in there in the first place, there would be nothing coming out.

I do not recommend that you do this for your child unless he or she is under the care of a health practitioner, as the heavy metals that potentially could be released can do a lot of immediate harm. If your child's pathways of elimination aren't open, the heavy metals will re-circulate and re-deposit, thereby potentially causing an acute health crisis.

Stool Test

A heavy metal stool test is ideal for monitoring the efficacy of natural detoxification of metals from your child's body and also for determining the level of dietary exposure to metals.

Blood Test

A blood test for heavy metals, like the one your pediatrician typically runs for your child to check for lead exposure, shows only acute levels of heavy metals that your child has been exposed to in the last 4 to 6 weeks. After that time, the metals get deposited and bound to tissues and organs in the body, so the true "body burden" of these metals won't be represented by the results of a blood test.

Electro-dermal Screening

My naturopath, Dr. Marvin Schweitzer, uses an ASYRA machine for electro-dermal screening, although there are other types out there. This type of screening is based on the principle that your body is made of energy. If you've ever had acupuncture done, you know that different organs and systems in your body have different energetic readings. The energy of the liver, for example, is different from the energy of the thyroid. Electro-dermal screening reads different energy systems in the body and can tell the practitioner whether organs or systems are out of balance.

I have no trouble accepting this premise because of the classes I took in remote sensing satellite imagery. In class, we learned that everything has a unique "spectral signature," giving off a unique combination of light wavelengths from far infrared, infrared, visible colors and ultraviolet light. For example, a remote-sensing satellite can tell that it's looking at a crop of wheat next to a maple-tree forest near a cold-water lake because each of these things reflects a unique pattern of light, which is energy. I think it's pretty much the same principle as electro-dermal screening. As with remote sensing, even non-living things like vitamins, minerals, hormones, and heavy metals can be "read" by these machines, which allow the practitioner to test different substances and foods in a person to see if they resonate. Sounds pretty "woo woo," doesn't it? But it works.

Testing for Pesticides, Carcinogens and Other Toxins

Although there may be other labs that test for pesticides, carcinogens and other toxins, I am not aware of them. Genova Diagnostics, which recently merged with MetaMetrix, offers a range of tests to check your child's exposure:

- Chlorinated pesticides profile – serum
- Phthalates and parabens profile – urine

- Toxic effects CORE
- Toxic effects clearance profile
- Volatile solvents profile – whole blood

Testing for Radiation

Most people have not had acute exposure to radiation from an accident or attack. Rather, we are exposed to low levels of it chronically. Radiation bioaccumulates, too, just as other environmental toxins do, so what counts is the chronic and consistent exposure to it. Other than scanning your child with a Geiger counter, the only alternatives I've come across for checking radiation in your child are electro-dermal screening and medical intuitives.

Gut Dysbiosis

Many, if not all, neurological disorders such as Sensory Processing Disorder, autism, PDD-NOS, ADHD, depression, schizophrenia, bipolar disorder and multiple sclerosis have gut dysbiosis as a core, underlying feature. It's also present in digestive disorders such as acid reflux, colic, colitis, Crohn's, celiac and eosiniphilic espohagitis as well as in autoimmune diseases such as rheumatoid arthritis, fibromyalgia and lupus.

What is gut dysbiosis? It's where the balance of flora in the intestine is tipped towards having more "bad" bacteria, yeasts and parasites than "good," It boils down to this: 70% of your child's immune system is located in their gut. If the inner ecosystem is overrun by bad guys, like *Candida*, it can leave your child vulnerable to more virulent infections, diseases and disorders.

The reason why gut dysbiosis plays such an important role in your child's sensory issues is due to the gut-brain connection, as documented by Michael Gershon, MD in *The Second Brain: A Groundbreaking New Understanding of Nervous Disorders of the Stomach and Intestine.* Most neurotransmitters are made in the gut, so if the gut isn't happy, the brain isn't happy.

The intestinal tract is a critical route for the elimination of toxins. A gut that is chronically constipated can't perform this important task. In addition, certain kinds of gut bacteria are essential for detoxifying the body, especially from mercury.[113]

Symptoms of Gut Dysbiosis

See if your child has any of these symptoms; they can be indicative of gut dysbiosis:

- One or two red cheeks after eating
- Red or hot ears after eating
- Chronic runny nose or cough
- Recurrent ear infections
- Chronic or recurrent sinus infections
- Chronic or recurrent strep infections
- Patches of red, dry, scaly skin (eczema) on face, hands, elbows, knees or other parts of the skin
- Frequent diaper rashes in babies
- Cradle cap or excessive scaling and dandruff on the scalp
- Dark circles or bags surrounding the eyes, "droopy" eyes (allergic shiners)
- Excessive drooling in children too old to drool
- Frequent temper tantrums
- Colic, excessive crying or irritability in babies
- Acid reflux
- Chronic spitting up or regurgitating after eating
- Arching the back and screaming when a baby is placed flat
- White coating on the tongue (thrush)
- Chronic thrush infections
- Unusual fingernail or toenail formation
- Chronic constipation
- Chronic diarrhea
- Chronic tummy aches

---

113. Rowland, I.R., et al, Effects of diet on mercury metabolism and excretion in mice given methylmercury: role of gut flora, *Arch Environ Health.* 1984 Nov-Dec;39(6):401-8.

- Distended "pot belly"
- Persistent aggressive behavior
- Persistent non-compliant or oppositional behavior
- Tics (verbal or physical) (including constant throat clearing, coughing, blinking)
- Recurrent urinary tract infections
- Chronic vaginal infections
- Chronic athletes foot, ring worm or other fungal skin infections[114]

Gut dysbiosis can also cause mental health issues such as depression, anxiety, bipolar disorder, schizophrenia and obsessive/compulsive disorder (OCD). This may not make much sense to you until you understand that a lot of serotonin – the neurotransmitter that makes you feel happy – is produced in the gut. When the gut's function is impaired, such as by gut dysbiosis, it's going to affect whether or not you feel good.

My older son had a far longer list of these symptoms than my younger one: recurrent ear infections, eczema, cradle cap, allergic shiners, frequent temper tantrums, acid reflux, constipation, a delay in walking – he was TWENTY months old – large motor delays, sensory defensiveness, failure to thrive, hypotonia, and extreme fatigue. My younger son had a shorter list: eczema, bloody diaper rashes, acid reflux, and a delay in walking (he was 16 months old).

I didn't even start to realize until my older son was four years old and my younger son was two what was going on with them. The person that helped me recover them the most certainly wasn't any of their pediatricians or allergist or gastroenterologist. When I started seeing a naturopath, Dr. Marvin Schweitzer, for my own health problems, I began to understand that the causes of my own health problems were

114. http://www.epidemicanswers.org/symptoms/soft-signs/ Accessed September 28, 2014.

the same causes of my children's, and gut dysbiosis played a huge role in all of our health problems.

Causes of Gut Dysbiosis

Most people don't understand how the use of steroids, antibiotics, birth-control pills and even ibuprofen can negatively affect the gut's ecosystem. The Standard American Diet (SAD) with its grain, sugar and starches also contributes heavily to a disrupted gut ecology. Many things can cause gut dysbiosis, among them:

- Inheriting it from your mother because she had gut dysbiosis when she gave birth to you.
- Inheriting it from your mother because she received antibiotics while she was in labor with you.
- Taking antibiotics.
- Taking birth-control pills.
- Taking cortisone or other steroids.
- Taking NSAIDs (non-steroidal anti-inflammatory drugs) such as ibuprofen and aspirin.
- Drinking chlorinated water.
- Using anti-bacterial soap or sanitizer.
- Eating added sugar or sweeteners.
- Eating processed foods such as breads, cereals, crackers, cookies, pastries, cakes and candy because they essentially break down into sugar and/or have high levels of added sugar.
- Eating too many fruits.
- Eating too much high-glycemic fruit such as tropical fruits like bananas, mangos and pineapples and dried fruits. Dried fruits, like raisins and dates, have very high concentrations of sugar.
- Eating vinegar and vinegar-brined foods.
- Eating non-organic meats from animals that have been given antibiotics. Remember, your child eats what they eat.

- Stress.
- Living in a damp or moldy environment.

Passed from Mother to Child

A mother can pass gut dysbiosis unknowingly on to her child. This is more likely if the mother was given antibiotics during labor, has a history of vaginal yeast infections and/or a history of taking birth-control pills, antibiotics or steroids. For example, mom can unknowingly have Lyme disease before or during pregnancy then pass it on to her baby. Lyme disease can be a hidden source of neurodevelopmental damage in children, as we'll go over later in the book.

Candida Overgrowth

The simplest way for me to think of gut dysbiosis is that it generally is caused by chronic and/or systemic yeast (usually *Candida albicans*) overgrowth. A research study by Rice University showed that 70% of people have an overgrowth of the *Candida albicans* fungus.[115] Yeast loves to eat sugar, so anything that breaks down too easily into sugar feeds the yeast and can cause it to grow to an unhealthy proportion. Also, anything that kills off bacteria (such as antibiotics, chlorinated water and anti-inflammatory drugs) causes collateral damage by killing all the "good" bacteria, too.

As Dr. William Crook discussed in his *Yeast Connection* books, many chronic issues are due to a buildup of yeast (*Candida*) in the body. Because many doctors don't offer systemic *Candida* infections as a diagnosis, it is often overlooked as a causative factor in autoimmune, neurological and hormonal diseases, disorders and conditions, even cancer, when, in my mind, it should be one of the first suspects.

Not only that, but *Candida* can affect your child's ability to

115. Ullmann, B.D., et al, Inducible defense mechanism against nitric oxide in Candida albicans, *Eukaryot Cell.* 2004 Jun;3(3):715-23.

produce hormones, which is why people with candidiasis often have adrenal, thyroid and reproductive-hormone problems. People with candidiasis are frequently fatigued, get sick a lot, have "female problems," food allergies, chemical sensitivities, constant headaches and other symptoms that are often dismissed by the medical establishment.

In its proper proportion, *Candida albicans* is actually a helpful yeast because it aids in digestion and the absorption of nutrients. It's just that when it grows out of control that it can cause problems such as ear and sinus infections, yeast infections, fatigue, brain fog, and mood swings. It can also cause a leaky gut because the yeast overgrowth props open the walls of the intestine, letting out undigested food. This creates inflammation throughout the body in the form of allergies, arthritis and other autoimmune diseases, fatigue and brain fog. Gluten and casein, if leaked out, travel through the bloodstream into the brain and cause a morphine-like effect, making it seem sometimes as if your child is on drugs when he or she eats these foods.

Antibiotics

The use of antibiotics is well-documented in the medical literature for its ability to cause gut dysbiosis. Overuse of antibiotics not only promotes the development of drug-resistant strains of bacteria but also leads to immune dysregulation.[116] Even one treatment with antibiotics can disrupt a baby's immune system.[117] Even if your child never received antibiotics, if the child's mother or grandmother did, then disrupted gut flora gets passed onto to the baby during birth.

If your child is eating non-organic meats, there's a good

---

116. Blaser, M., Antibiotic overuse: Stop the killing of beneficial bacteria, *Nature*, 476, 393–394 (25 August 2011).
117. Ambrose, N.S., The influence of single dose intravenous antibiotics on faecal flora and emergence of Clostridium difficile, *J Antimicrob Chemother.* 1985 Mar;15(3):319-26.

chance those animals were grown with antibiotics. Feed-lot animals are typically grown in pens so tight they can't even turn around. Because of this, these animals are highly stressed and get sick a lot, which is why they're given a lot of antibiotics.

Sugar, Grains and Starches

Sugar, even sugar from dairy products, as well as all types of sugar such as maple syrup, rice syrup and high-fructose corn syrup, feeds parasites and pathogens in the gut. In addition, grains and starches can contribute to gut dysbiosis if they are not combined properly with proteins and protein-fats like avocados, seeds, nuts and olives. Think about the foods that your children eat; they are typically very sugar and processed-carb heavy.

Acidic pH

An acidic pH below 7.0 encourages the growth of parasites and pathogens in the gut. Sugar is the most acidic food, and meat is close behind. An acidic gut is typically anaerobic, meaning there's not much oxygen in there, and this is a perfect environment for gut dysbiosis.

Birthing Practices

One of the reasons why we're seeing such an increase in children's chronic health conditions is because more and more women are having C-sections; fully one third of all babies in America are delivered via C-section. Sometimes this is due to fetal induction, sometimes it's due to multiple births, and sometimes it's just more convenient for the doctor and/or mother. If a woman has a C-section, antibiotics are administered, and the baby doesn't receive any flora, good or bad, from her birth canal. Instead, it picks up only what's floating around the hospital.

In addition, many times during childbirth, women are

given antibiotic drips prophylactically because they have mitral valve prolapse or tested positive for strep B. The thing is, most people have strep B bacteria on them. Whether or not you get an infection from it is determined by the immune system.

Feeding Practices

Breastfeeding is another way to transfer not only healthy flora on to your baby but also important immune-system supportive nutrients. However, according to the CDC, although 76.5% of mothers began breastfeeding their babies at birth, only 16.4% were exclusively breastfeeding at six months.[118] Infant formula not only doesn't contain beneficial flora, but it is also loaded with ingredients such as corn syrup solids and soy protein isolates, sugar and vegetable oil that contribute to gut dysbiosis and poor health.

Researchers from the Touro College of Osteopathic Medicine discovered that breastfeeding may help prevent autism because breast milk contains insulin-like growth factor (IGF), which promotes the development of myelin, an insulating material, around developing nerves.[119] Myelin is essential for the efficient transmission of brain signals in functions such as thinking, emotions and sensory perception.

Bacterial Infections

In addition to *Candida* overgrowth, many children with Sensory Processing Disorder, as well as other neurodevelopmental disorders, often have bacterial infections in the gut. *Clostridia (C. difficile)*, *Klebsiella*, and *Streptococcus* are common bacterial infections.

---

118. http://www.cdc.gov/breastfeeding/pdf/2013breastfeedingreportcard.pdf. Accessed September 13, 2014.
119. Steinman, G., et al, Breastfeeding as a possible deterrent to autism--a clinical perspective, *Med Hypotheses.* 2013 Dec;81(6):999-1001.

Parasites

Americans and people from other Western cultures seem to think that parasitic infections are a developing world problem. This isn't the case, as Ann Louise Gittleman, PhD, CNS, points out in *Guess What Came to Dinner?: Parasites and Your Health.* She says that Americans host up to 130 different kinds of parasites and that one person in six is infected with them.[120] *Giardia lamblia*, a water-borne parasite, is the most common culprit.

Viral Infections

Viruses might also be hanging out in your child's tummy, especially if there's a biofilm slime surrounding it. The measles, rubella, chickenpox, mumps, cytomegalovirus and herpes simplex viruses have all been associated with autism.[121]

Lyme Disease

Lyme disease isn't just infection from the Lyme spirochete bacterium. There are also co-infections – *Bartonella, Babesia* and *Erlichia* – that typically may occur at the same time. Or someone could just get one of the co-infections without having any of the other co-infections of Lyme. Lyme can masquerade not only as autism and developmental delays but also as rheumatoid arthritis (RA), fibromyalgia, multiple sclerosis and neurological damage. In my mind, it should be one of the first things tested for when an autoimmune disease or neurological dysfunction has a sudden onset. It's becoming a hidden epidemic, as not a lot of doctors know to test for it.

There's an excellent documentary about Lyme called

---

120. Gittleman, Ann Louise, *Guess What Came to Dinner?: Parasites and Your Health.* New York, NY: Penguin Putnam Inc., 2001, 7.
121. Libbey, J.E., Autistic disorder and viral infections, *J Neurovirol.* 2005 Feb;11(1):1-10.

Under Our Skin. I specifically remember a beautiful woman documented in the film who became increasingly contorted. She gradually lost control of many of her muscles, and doctors thought she had multiple sclerosis (MS). The reason that we know it wasn't MS is that she regained her strength and control after a very long course of antibiotics, so it was obviously an infection. How many people that have Sensory Processing Disorder, MS, RA, fibromyalgia, autism or developmental delays simply have Lyme or a co-infection? It's a real shame they're not getting proper treatment.

Lyme is not just limited to the Northeastern U.S. anymore; it's now spreading west to places where you wouldn't think deer ticks are. Deer ticks are not the only means of transmission: mosquitoes, fleas and other ticks can also carry the infection. Given that there is an increasing number of people with gut dysbiosis and toxicity, and thus, a compromised immune system, it's not surprising that their weakened state allows for such an infection.

Lymedisease.org lists the following common symptoms of children with Lyme:

- Headache
- Stiff neck
- Light or sound sensitivity
- Cognitive impairment
- Uncharacteristic behavior
- Inability to sustain attention
- Outbursts & mood swings
- Arthritis
- Fatigue
- Abdominal pain, nausea, diarrhea
- Chest pain, palpitations
- Shortness of breath
- Night sweats

- Tingling, burning or shooting pains[122]

Could this be your SPD child? Lymedisease.org says that 50% of children with Lyme have no history of tick attachment and that less than 70% of people develop the classic "bull's-eye" rash. Lyme can get passed from mother to child, as many infections can. Personally, I know a few moms who passed it on to their children; these children have autism, ADHD and/or Sensory Processing Disorder.

Here a few other symptoms in children:

- Hypotonia
- Clumsiness
- Learning disabilities
- Vision problems
- Fear of heights
- Rages
- OCD
- Heartburn
- Achiness, especially in the knees

Testing for Lyme Disease

Lyme disease and its co-infections are difficult to test for. One reason is due to the corkscrew shape of the bacteria, which allows them to burrow in without being easily detected. Spirochetes (see the word "spiral" in there?) are one of the most ancient forms of life on this Earth, and they know how to survive and adapt to rapidly changing environments.

Most doctors will run a simple lab test, but it's not sensitive enough; it misses too many cases. Igenex's test is more advanced, more sensitive and looks for more genuses. Dietrich Klinghardt, MD, PhD, a Lyme-literate doctor, suggests the following are indicative of a Lyme infection:

---

122. http://lymedisease.org/lyme101/lyme_disease/children_symptoms.html. Accessed September 12, 2014.

- Low white blood count
- Elevated MCV
- Elevated fasting blood sugar
- Moderately elevated LDL with low cholesterol and low triglycerides
- Low urine specific gravity
- Very low triglycerides with low cholesterol
- Low alkaline phosphatase[123]

You can ask your doctor to work with you on getting more sensitive tests for your child such as an Igenex Western blot.

Lyme Disease: A Case Study

When my older son was six, he had a definite change in his typically sweet personality for the worst. Given that he already been recovered from Sensory Processing Disorder, I was confused. This time, he was ANGRY. In fact, every time I would ask him to do something, he would yell back at me and say that I hated him and that I was yelling, when in fact I wasn't yelling at all. Almost every day he would look at me with total hatred and anger, stomp out the front door and tell me he was running away from home. I was really confused because these were supposed to be the "golden" years of childhood when there's not so much hands-on work to do with children this age and they are happy to be with their family. I kept thinking "If he's like this as a child, what the heck is he going to be like as a teenager?" This went on for a while until I remembered about Lyme disease. Lyme disease can cause sudden changes in behavior, and we live in tick-ridden Connecticut, so this wasn't a far-out hypothesis.

My son's uncharacteristic behavior, outbursts and mood swings really made me suspect that it might be Lyme. I did more research on it, especially about Dr. Charles Ray Jones, a Lyme pediatric specialist who practices near my town. I had

---

123. Klinghardt, Dietrich, MD, PhD. *Healing the Brain* conference, New York, NY, May 2013.

heard him speak before at Dietrich Klinghardt's Klinghardt Academy in New York City a few months prior; Dr. Klinghardt also specializes in difficult-to-treat disorders, like Lyme, autism and autoimmune diseases. Dr. Jones is fairly famous in the Lyme disease community for recovering children from what is thought to be Sensory Processing Disorder, autism, ADHD, OCD, ODD and other neurodevelopmental disorders. It turns out that in MANY of these cases, these children actually had Lyme disease. Dr. Jones has recovered over 10,000 children from these disorders. He prescribes various antibiotics for a course of many years, whereas if you were to go to a typical doctor for treatment of Lyme, he or she would prescribe antibiotics for a few weeks or months.

Personally, I wouldn't want to subject myself or my children to antibiotics for any amount of time these days, knowing what I know about how they destroy the immune system. But, hey, the man gets results, and the results show that many of these disorders are, in fact, from Lyme infections. In his presentation, he gave a few examples of children. One of them was a young boy who at a very young age of six had already been in and out of juvenile detention for things like harming animals, which is a known sign of a child or person on the road to becoming a hardened criminal. After a few months of treatment from Dr. Jones, this same boy had become the sweetest, most likeable child.

Dr. Jones typically suspects Lyme if the child has any of the following conditions:

- Frequent fever
- Increased incidence of throat and ear infections
- Increased incidence of pneumonia
- Irritability
- Joint and body pain
- Hypotonia
- Acid reflux
- Small windpipe (tracheomalacia)
- Cataracts and other eye problems
- Developmental delays

- Learning disabilities
- Psychiatric problems

What's interesting is that 50% of Dr. Jones' patients have no known history of being bitten by a deer tick and fewer than 10% have the classic Lyme bull's-eye rash (erythema migrans). In fact, many times the mother unknowingly passed the infection on to the child during pregnancy or childbirth.

Given the confusion surrounding the issue of detecting Lyme, I asked our naturopath to test my son for Lyme with his ASYRA. Sure enough, my son was infected with *Bartonella*, also known as cat-scratch fever. Rather than going the antibiotics route, our naturopath prescribed a super-strong herbal remedy. A couple of months after treatment, my son was no longer hateful or hurtful and is now the super-sweet boy I remember.

Testing for Gut Dysbiosis

There are many tests available that can test for gut dysbiosis; the trick is to find a practitioner that uses them. Typical ones are:

- Comprehensive digestive stool analysis (CDSA)
- Organic acids test (OAT)
- Small intestine bacterial overgrowth (SIBO)

Immune Dysregulation

The body of a child with a dysregulated immune system cannot appropriately respond to environmental triggers. Autoimmunity is a classic example of this because a person with this kind of disorder has an immune system that is always on the attack, so much so, that it is attacking itself. Any child with a leaky gut is likely to have immune dysregulation because waste that should be pooped out sometimes recirculates into the body, causing the body to attack itself.

What's important to understand is what is meant by "autoimmune". Most people think of it as the classic examples of autoimmune such as lupus, multiple sclerosis, rheumatoid arthritis, scleroderma and fibromyalgia, but it should also be understood as any condition in which the body has an allergic reaction, too, such as allergies, eczema and asthma.

Symptoms of Immune Dysregulation

A dysregulated immune system is one that responds inappropriately. Some SPD kids have overactive immune systems, while those of others cannot mount a sufficient immune response. Some of the symptoms of immune dysregulation are:

- Autoimmune symptoms
- Chronic inflammation
- Chronic allergies
- A child who is always sick
- A child who is never sick

Causes of Immune Dysregulation

Toxicity, gut dysbiosis, sugar, stress and maternal inheritance are the major causes of immune dysregulation.

Toxicity

Toxins are foreign substances in the body, and they cause chronic inflammation. Because toxins aren't being flushed from the body by peeing, pooping, sweating and breathing, the body responds to toxins such as heavy metals, EMFs and endocrine disruptors by going on the attack.

Gut Dysbiosis

Why is gut dysbiosis such a bad thing? It causes immune

dysfunction. Did you know that 70% of the immune system is actually in the gut? If the gut isn't working properly, neither is the immune system. All of those pounds of flora, good and bad, in the gut are communicating with the immune-system cells in the gut and telling them whether or not to turn on certain genetic switches. If your child has the wrong kind of flora (bad bacteria, yeast overgrowth, viral infection or parasitic invasion) telling his or her genes what to do, your child is going to end up in bad health. It's like having your kids hang out with the wrong crowd; you know they're going to end up in trouble. Dysbiosis can lead to a weakened immune system, which can make the body more hospitable to parasites and infectious invasion.

Sugar

Sugar suppresses the immune system. Glucose, fructose, sucrose and other simple sugars cause a 50% reduction in the number of white blood cells that engulf pathogenic bacteria.[124]

Stress

Stress can definitely dysregulate the immune system. It causes undue strain on the adrenals and thyroid, causes inflammation, disrupts the gut microbiome and steals nutrients. Have you ever gotten a cold after burning out dealing with a stressful event? That's an example of stress causing immune dysregulation.

Passed from Mother to Child

Researchers discovered that a maternal history of autoimmune disease "was significantly associated with a modest increase in odds of developmental disorders" including

---

124. http://www.askdrsears.com/topics/feeding-eating/family-nutrition/sugar/harmful-effects-excess-sugar. Accessed September 1, 2014.

autism but that it's likely not the only causative factor.[125] Many moms of children with Sensory Processing Disorder, autism, ADHD and other chronic disorders have a history of lupus, allergies, asthma, multiple sclerosis, rheumatoid arthritis or other autoimmune conditions on their side of the family.

Nutritional Deficiencies

Deficiencies of critical nutrients is a given in a child with Sensory Processing Disorder, as well as in any person with a chronic disease. These children are typically deficient in a variety of nutrients such as vitamin D, vitamin B_{12}, essential fatty acids and key minerals. I'll address these specific nutrients later in the chapter.

Causes of Nutritional Deficiencies

Toxicity, gut dysbiosis and poor diet are common causes of deficiencies. Other causes are deficiencies passed from mother to child, modern agricultural practices, low stomach acid, low levels of pancreatic enzymes, birthing practices and picky eating.

Toxicity

If you read *Detoxify or Die* by Sherry Rogers, MD, you'll get a sense for just how much toxicity causes nutritional deficiencies. The liver needs extra nutrients to detoxify these poisons, and the body in general needs extra nutrients such as antioxidants, vitamins and minerals to lower inflammation caused by them as well.

---

125. Lyall, K., Maternal immune-mediated conditions, autism spectrum disorders, and developmental delay, *J Autism Dev Disord.* 2014 Jul;44(7):1546-55.

Pharmaceuticals

Sherry Rogers, MD says that pharmaceuticals poison nutritional pathways to create deficiencies. Suzy Cohen, RPh, calls them "drug muggers," in her book, *Drug Muggers: Which Medications Are Robbing Your Body of Essential Nutrients—and Natural Ways to Restore Them.* The point is that the liver needs extra nutrients to detoxify from the pharmaceuticals, and these drugs rob your child's body of critical nutrients that he or she is likely already deficient in. In fact, pharmaceuticals merely suppress symptoms of a disease or disorder. Many times, these symptoms are created by nutritional deficiencies, so putting your child on any kind of pharmaceutical can cause a downward spiral of greater nutrient deficiency.

Passed from Mother to Child

I had a great "aha!" moment when I read Julia Ross's book, *The Mood Cure: The 4-Step Program to Take Control of Your Emotions— Today.* She is well-known for her use of amino acid therapy in the recovery of alcoholics and drugs addicts. In her latest book, *The Diet Cure: The 8-Step Program to Rebalance Your Body Chemistry and End Food Cravings, Weight Gain, and Mood Swings— Naturally*, she writes how women become nutritionally deficient after years and even decades of dieting. A woman eating low-fat, no-fat food is by default likely eating a high-carbohydrate diet and is also likely not eating enough protein. Guess where amino acids come from? Protein.

The "aha!" came when I thought about all of these women going on to have babies: they're passing on their nutritional deficiencies, including amino-acid deficiencies. All those women that have been on nutritionally deficient diets for years since at least the 1970s are having kids, and those kids are being born with nutritional deficiencies that are compounded by gut dysbiosis, toxicity and stress. No wonder we're seeing such epidemics of Sensory Processing Disorder, autism, ADHD, allergies and more. Moms being on nutritionally deficient diets isn't the only reason for this epidemic, but it certainly plays a key, overlooked role.

Modern Agricultural Practices

Because of modern growing practices, the foods we eat today are woefully deficient in minerals. Farmers today practice monoculture, use synthetic fertilizers and pesticides, and don't allow fields to lie fallow, which would increase the amount of nutrients in the soil. All of these practices strip minerals from an already deficient soil. In addition, the application of pesticides can allow crops to grow faster than they normally would, which allows the crop less time to absorb nutrients from the soil.

Standard American Diet (SAD)

In addition to containing GMO foods, the Standard American Diet typically contains health-damaging "foods" such as vegetable oils, trans fats, artificial colors, artificial flavors, "natural" flavors, preservatives, artificial sweeteners, flavor enhancers and other additives that typically haven't been studied for safety. Many of these additives are toxic, as I've shown you, while others such as sugar, high-fructose corn syrup and low-fat/non-fat foods are nutrient-poor and/or create further deficiencies.

Sugar

Sugar is pushed on us by an agricultural policy that subsidizes corn and sugar, making it a cheap and addictive additive to processed foods. I think by now, we all know that sugar and processed foods can lead to diabetes and obesity, but sugar also uses up valuable nutrients to process it. For example, it takes a LOT of magnesium to process sugar, and magnesium is both woefully deficient in the Standard American Diet and necessary to calm the central nervous system. In addition, sugar increases your child's appetite. Sugar doesn't tell your child's brain that it's full and that they should stop eating, which is why they can scarf down a whole box of crackers or cookies and still be hungry. Sugar therefore causes your child to eat a lot of nutrient-deficient food.

High-Fructose Corn Syrup

High-fructose corn syrup is almost always a marker for nutritionally deficient processed food. For example, soda is loaded with sugar in the form of high-fructose corn syrup. A 12-ounce can of soda contains 39 grams of sugar. That's equivalent to over 3 TABLESPOONS of sugar per drink.

High fructose corn syrup also contains toxic amounts of mercury; your child receives the equivalent of receiving two fillings per day by eating the amount that the typical American does per day.[126] Chlor-alkali products used in the manufacture of high-fructose corn syrup leaves behind toxic amounts of mercury, a known neurotoxin, and toxins create nutritional deficiencies.

Low-Fat or Non-Fat Food

It is my belief that the rise of low-fat and non-fat foods in the past few decades is responsible for the epidemics of obesity, heart disease and diabetes because they are by default higher in sugar and lower in fat. Fat is not the enemy, unless it's vegetable oils or trans fats. Instead, the enemy is sugar, which is the most inflammatory food. Fat sends a satiety signal to your child's brain, sugar does not, and a high-carb/high-sugar/low-fat diet can cause blood-sugar swings in your SPD child.

---

126. Rogers, Sherry, MD, *Total Wellness Newsletter*, February 2014, 3.

Low Stomach Acid

A child with low stomach acid cannot properly digest his or her food. Proteins won't get completely broken down into amino acids, and minerals and vitamin B_{12} won't be pulled out, leading to dangerous deficiencies of critical nutrients. Stress, infection and acid-reflux medications such as proton-pump inhibitors like Prevacid® and Prilosec® as well as acid blockers like Tums® are the most common causes of low stomach acid.

Gut Dysbiosis

Pathogens and parasites in the gut rob your child's body of critical nutrients. The intestinal tract's job is to absorb nutrients, but if there is dysbiosis, the digestive and absorptive processes are likely compromised.

Cord Clamping

Many of the common practices in pregnancy, childbirth and infant care are driven, many times without safety studies, to keep you and your baby as a profit center. Cord clamping is an example of such a practice. Instead of letting critical nutrients take their time to flow from you to your newborn after birth – sometimes, this can take hours – the baby's umbilical cord is almost immediately clamped because a hospital's goal is to get you processed as quickly as they can. A recent study concluded that "delayed cord clamping has been associated with decreased iron-deficient anemia and increased iron stores with potential valuable effects that extend beyond the newborn period, including improvements in long-term neurodevelopment."[127]

---

127. McAdams, R.M., Time to implement delayed cord clamping, *Obstet Gynecol.* 2014 Mar;123(3):549-52.

Picky Eating

Children with Sensory Processing Disorder, autism, ADHD, allergies, asthma, learning disabilities and developmental delays are often picky eaters. Typically, this is caused by nutritional deficiencies, and picky eating can compound these deficiencies. Picky eaters are the kids that will only eat "white" foods: cheese pizza, chicken nuggets, crackers, chips, yogurt and the like. The Standard American Diet's "white" foods have a lot to do with creating picky eaters that prefer the taste of artificially flavored processed foods over whole foods, but there's more to it: nutritional deficiencies get passed from mother to child. So typically, where there's a picky child, there's often a mom who's either a picky eater herself or who's dieted quite a bit in her life.

It's hard to get these kids to eat vegetables or whole foods, which is a shame, because these are the kinds of foods that can help correct nutritional deficiencies. In my experience, MOST kids these days are picky eaters. I never cease to be shocked at the eating habits of kids and how little variety they eat. Then again, 54% of kids these days have some form of chronic illness.[128]

Types of Deficiencies

There are many deficiencies that are common in children with Sensory Processing Disorder: magnesium, zinc, iodine, iron, vitamin D, fatty acids, glutathione, stomach acid, methylated nutrients, amino acids, melatonin and pancreatic enzymes. Not every child will be deficient in all of these, so please don't assume that your child is; in addition, because every child is different, your child may have a completely different set of deficiencies. You need to have them tested, which I will cover later in the chapter.

---

128. Bethell, C.D., et al, A national and state profile of leading health problems and health care quality for US children: key insurance disparities and across-state variations, *Acad Pediatr.* 2011 May-Jun;11(3 Suppl):S22-33.

Magnesium Deficiency

As much as 80% of Americans are deficient in magnesium, which is a vital mineral for our hearts, bones, gut health, nervous system, sugar metabolism and so much more. SPD kids have a higher-than-normal need for it because of the stress of not being able to process their senses correctly and because of underlying toxicity. It's a sad fact that our soils are depleted of minerals from over-farming, non-crop rotation and heavy use of pesticides, so even if your child is eating a vegetable-rich diet (one of the main sources of magnesium), he or she is likely not getting near enough magnesium for optimal health. Add to that the fact that many pharmaceuticals such as painkillers, acid-reflux medication, antibiotics, diuretics and cortisone deplete magnesium as do our stressful and processed-food lifestyles.

It's no wonder, then, that magnesium is a miracle mineral, as Dr. Carolyn Dean writes about in her book, *The Magnesium Miracle*. She writes that a magnesium deficiency is linked to:

- Anxiety and panic attacks
- Asthma
- Blood clots
- Bowel disease
- Cystitis
- Depression
- Diabetes
- Dysmenorrhea
- Fatigue
- Heart disease
- Hypertension
- Hypoglycemia
- Inability to detoxify
- Insomnia
- Kidney disease
- Liver disease
- Migraines
- Musculoskeletal conditions

- Nerve problems
- Premenstrual syndrome
- Osteoporosis
- Raynaud's Syndrome
- Tooth decay[129]

Dr. Dean calls magnesium the "spark of life" because it is so essential for so many bodily functions.[130] As a doctor, she believes that other doctors should make it one of their first treatment options.

Zinc Deficiency

Picky eaters with poor appetites are often zinc deficient. Zinc not only improves your child's sense of taste and smell, but also is necessary for the thyroid and immune system, two critical components of Sensory Processing Disorder. Other symptoms of low zinc levels are low muscle tone and white spots or lines on your child's fingernails.

Iodine Deficiency

Dr. David Brownstein in his book, *Iodine: Why You Need It, Why You Can't Live Without It*, says that 92% of his patients initially show iodine deficiency, which he then explains is a major cause of breast and ovarian cancers, as well as hypothyroidism and ADHD.[131] SPD kids are typically hypothyroid, as I'll discuss later in this chapter.

---

129. Dean, Carolyn, MD, ND, *The Magnesium Miracle* . New York, NY: Ballantine Books, 2007, xviii-xxi.
130. Ibid, p. 12.
131. Brownstein, David, MD, *Iodine: Why You Need It, Why You Can't Live Without It.* West Bloomfield, MI: Medical Alternative Press, 2009, 49.

Iron Deficiency

Iron deficiency is often seen in children with neurodevelopmental disorders. For example, children with autism under the age of six tend to have anemia more often than their older counterparts. This may have something to do malabsorption and a less-mature gastrointestinal tract.[132] In addition, iron deficiency is often linked to ADHD symptoms. Premature babies given supplemental iron are less likely to develop ADHD later in life.[133] NEVER give your child iron without testing and the advice of a doctor, however, as iron overdose is one of the leading causes of death in children under the age of six.

Vitamin D Deficiency

Vitamin D is notoriously low in children with autism,[134] and there is a vitamin D deficiency epidemic in most other people, too, these days. Laila Y. Al-Ayadh, head researcher of a study about deficiency of vitamin D in children with autism, says that, "There is a growing body of literature linking vitamin D to various immune-related conditions, including allergy and autoimmunity."[135]

Sunlight is necessary to convert the cholesterol in your child's skin to vitamin D, and if he or she isn't playing outside enough or lives in low-sunlight areas, he or she will be

---

132. Reynolds, A., et al, Iron status in children with autism spectrum disorder, *Pediatrics*. 2012 Nov;130 Suppl 2:S154-9.

133. Berglund, S.K., et al, Effects of Iron Supplementation of LBW Infants on Cognition and Behavior at 3 Years, *Pediatrics*, Dec. 10 2012

134. Neggers, Y.H., Increasing prevalence, changes in diagnostic criteria, and nutritional risk factors for autism spectrum disorders, *ISRN Nutr.* 2014 Feb 13;2014:514026.

135. Mostafa, G.A., et al, Reduced serum concentrations of 25-hydroxy vitamin D in children with autism: relation to autoimmunity, *J Neuroinflammation.* 2012 Aug 17;9:201.

deficient. People with darker skin are more at risk of being deficient in vitamin D.[136]

In addition, most people still believe that fats are bad for them, when in fact, fats are extremely healing. They are necessary for the activation of the fat-soluble vitamins A, D, E and K, and often contain them. Maybe the recent trend of eating low-fat foods is one of the many causes behind the epidemic of diseases that we're seeing these days. In addition, vitamin D is necessary for a healthy immune system because it regulates the gut microbiome.[137]

Essential Fatty Acid Deficiencies

Children with neurodevelopmental disorders are infamously deficient in essential fatty acids, likely due to mothers not breastfeeding them and due to eating the Standard American diet full of processed vegetable oils and trans fats. In fact, children who are not breastfed and who are deficient in essential fatty acids are more likely to have autism,[138] ADHD[139] and other neurodevelopmental disorders.

Glutathione Deficiency

Decreased levels of glutathione, the body's master antioxidant, are another hallmark of neurodevelopmental disorders such as autism,[140] ADHD[141] and other

---

136. Glover, T.L., Vitamin D, race, and experimental pain sensitivity in older adults with knee osteoarthritis, *Arthritis Rheum.* 2012 Dec;64(12):3926-35.
137. Ooi, J.H., et al, Vitamin D regulates the gut microbiome and protects mice from dextran sodium sulfate-induced colitis, *J Nutr.* 2013 Oct;143(10):1679-86.
138. Brown, C.M., et al, Observable essential fatty acid deficiency markers and autism spectrum disorder, *Breastfeed Rev.* 2014 Jul;22(2):21-6.
139. Quintero, J., et al, [Nutritional aspects of attention-deficit/hyperactive disorder], *Rev Neurol.* 2009 Sep 16-30;49(6):307-12.
140. Hodgson, N.W., et al, Decreased glutathione and elevated hair mercury levels are associated with nutritional deficiency-based autism in Oman, *Exp Biol Med* (Maywood). 2014 Mar 27;239(6):697-706.

neurodevelopmental disorders. This is likely due to the oxidative stress effects of toxicity and gut dysbiosis, as well as the use of Tylenol®, which is well known in its ability to lower glutathione. In fact, as shown earlier, the use of Tylenol® combined with vaccinations may be one of the leading causes of the rapid increase in the rate of neurodevelopmental disorders among children.

Stomach Acid Deficiency

Low stomach acid means that pathogenic yeast, bacteria and viruses can easily get through the stomach alive, which allows them to set up shop and colonize in the intestinal tract, causing dysbiosis. Many times, these critters create a biofilm in the gut that's impenetrable by antibiotics; the slimy biofilm steals important nutrients from your child's body while housing numerous pathogens. Care must be taken when implementing a biofilm protocol because when it starts to be destroyed by targeted supplements, live viruses and other pathogens are then freed to cause damage in your child's body.

Stomach acid is absolutely necessary to strip nutrients from food. A child who has low stomach acid typically is low in vitamin B_{12} and minerals. In addition, stomach acid is needed to pull apart protein into its constituent amino acids. Therefore, a child with low stomach acid is also typically deficient in key amino acids such as cysteine, glycine, tryptophan and carnitine.

Methyl Deficiencies

Methyl groups are found in methylated nutrients like methylcobalamin (vitamin B_{12}), methylfolate (vitamin B_9), methylated vitamin B_6 (pyridoxal 5-phosphate), methylated vitamin B_5 (riboflavin 5-phosphate sodium), trimethylglycine

141. Ceylan, M.F., et al, Changes in oxidative stress and cellular immunity serum markers in attention-deficit/hyperactivity disorder, *Psychiatry Clin Neurosci.* 2012 Apr;66(3):220-6.

(TMG) and dimethylglycine (DMG). Many children with Sensory Processing Disorder and other neurodevelopmental disorders typically have methyl deficiencies.

Methylation is the chemical process of donating a methyl group (CH_3) to a molecule or compound. This doesn't sound like much, but this little group is very important to how our bodies function. Methylation is an all-encompassing issue like toxicity or gut dysbiosis because so many diseases and conditions are linked, directly or indirectly, to it or rather, a lack of it.

Methylation not only helps with energy production and builds immune cells and neurotransmitters, but it also processes hormones, detoxifies the body, puts protective myelin sheath on the nerves, and can be responsible for epigenetic gene regulation.

MTHFR Mutation

Because of its association with all of these essential processes, an inability to methylate is linked to a whole host of diseases and conditions; this is known as an MTHFR (methyl tetrahydrofolate reductase) genetic mutation. Your child may have one or both of the common C677T or A1298C mutations. A genetic MTHFR mutation is one reason for a methylation defect, but there are several other causes of the defect, such as:

- Lack of cofactors: zinc, magnesium, or vitamin B_6
- Antacids
- Environmental toxicity

Methylation defects are linked to many common diseases and disorders, such as:

- Sensory Processing Disorder
- Diabetes
- Alcoholism
- Cardiovascular disease

- Cancer
- Osteoporosis
- Spina bifida
- Autism
- Fibromyalgia
- Pulmonary embolisms
- Cleft palette
- Parkinson's
- Neural tube defects
- Atherosclerosis
- Immune deficiency
- ADD/ADHD
- Multiple sclerosis
- Alzheimer's
- Dementia
- Chemical sensitivity
- Congenital heart defects
- Chronic fatigue syndrome
- Depression
- Addictive behaviors
- Insomnia
- Down's syndrome
- Chronic viral infection
- Thyroid dysfunction
- Neuropathy
- Recurrent miscarriages
- Infertility
- Anxiety
- Schizophrenia
- Allergies
- Asthma
- Bipolar disorder

Dr. Kenneth Bock's book, *Healing the New Childhood Epidemics: Autism, ADHD, Asthma, and Allergies: The Groundbreaking Program for the 4-A Disorders*, discusses what he calls the "miracle of methylation" in great detail. Many times, after taking methylated supplements or receiving methylocobalamin vitamin B_{12} shots, a child will begin speaking if he's had a language delay or show other big improvements in health and development.

Most, if not all, children with Sensory Processing Disorder, autism, ADHD, allergies and asthma have methylation defects and are therefore not able to eliminate toxins. So the toxins, especially heavy metals, accumulate and damage the nervous system, brain, tissues and organs.

Nutritionist Dr. Ann Louise Gittleman believes that the MTHFR gene is defective in nearly 30 – 50% of all Americans. She believes that it is the number one health problem in this country today. Benjamin Lynch, ND, who runs the MTHFR.net website, says that MTHFR defects are more common in white Europeans (25-45%) and U.S. Hispanics (42%), and less so in Asians (14%) and African Americans (14%).

Here's the tricky part, though. What we see listed as "folic acid" or "folate" on processed foods is not a high-dose methylated folate. It's a synthetic version that was mandated by the government back in the 1990's to help prevent birth defects. Synthetic folic acid (or just "folic acid" or "folate" on the label) can actually do MORE harm to people with a methylation defect because it causes their toxic load to accumulate rapidly. It also decreases natural killer cells, which are critical in fighting cancer.

According to the B_{12} Awareness website, a vitamin B_{12} deficiency is linked to multiple neurological disorders, including:

- Abnormal reflexes
- Anemia
- Anorexia
- Apathy
- Ataxia
- Balance problems
- Dementia
- Depression
- Developmental delays or regression

- Difficulty walking
- Dizziness
- Failure to thrive
- Fatigue
- Forgetfulness, memory loss
- Generalized weakness
- Hallucinations
- Hypotonia
- Impotence
- Involuntary movements
- Irritability
- Language delay
- Lower IQ
- Macrocytosis (enlarged red-blood cells)
- Mania
- Mental retardation
- Numbness or tingling
- Pallor
- Paranoia
- Personality changes
- Poor head growth
- Poor motor skills
- Poor socialization
- Poor weight gain
- Psychosis
- Restless legs
- Seizures
- Shortness of breath
- Speech problems
- Tremor
- Unsteady or abnormal gait
- Urinary or fecal incontinence
- Violent behavior
- Visual disturbances
- Weakness[142]

---

142. http://b12awareness.org/about-b12/signs-symptoms-neurologic-psychiatric-hematologic-infants-children/ Accessed September 14, 2014.

There are common causes to vitamin B_{12} deficiency, such as low stomach acid and anesthesia. I was upset when I learned about the role that anesthesia plays in lowering vitamin B_{12} because my younger son had a completely unnecessary endoscopy when he was a year old, just to confirm to the gastroenterologist and pediatrician that he did indeed have acid reflux, as I had been telling them for months. The nitrous oxide that the doctor gave my son to put him under depletes B_{12} reserves and can also lead to a dangerous B_{12} deficiency and neurological damage. After learning these things and after being dismissed and condescended to for so long by so many doctors, I really had had enough of allopathic doctors. Conventional, Western-style medicine is allopathic, and these types of doctors look at suppressing symptoms with either pharmaceuticals or surgery instead of trying to find out what is causing the symptom to begin with, such as dairy, in the cases of both of my sons.

Amino Acid Deficiencies

Many children with Sensory Processing Disorder are also deficient in some amino acids, such as glycine, cysteine, tryptophan, GABA and carnitine. Glycine and cysteine are used to make glutathione, tryptophan converts to serotonin and then melatonin, and glycine and GABA are also neurotransmitters. Deficiencies of them can cause anxiety and agitation. Carnitine is essential for fatty acid transport into the cells, and a deficiency of this is a hallmark of mitochondrial dysfunction, which will be discussed later in the book.

There are three main reasons for amino-acid deficiencies:

- Low stomach acid
- Low protein consumption, although I'm not advocating a high-protein diet
- Maternal deficiency

For example, a woman on Zoloft® or Prozac is likely

deficient in the amino acid tryptophan, which later gets converted into the serotonin neurotransmitter; therefore, her children are more likely to be tryptophan-deficient because she passes her deficiencies on to her children when she's pregnant with them.

Melatonin Deficiency

Children with neurodevelopmental disorders are infamous for their sleeping problems; this is likely due to deficiencies of magnesium, glycine – which helps your child to sleep through the night, GABA and melatonin. Children with neurodevelopmental disorders are very likely to be melatonin deficient,[143] likely because they have low stomach acid, gut dysbiosis, and possibly an inherited deficiency.

Melatonin is also a very powerful antioxidant, and the lack of it is one of the reasons behind the amount of inflammation in a child with Sensory Processing Disorder or other neurodevelopmental disorder.

Pancreatic Enzyme Deficiencies

Dr. Mark Sircus writes in *Sodium Bicarbonate - Full Medical Review* that the pancreas is the first organ to develop inhibited function from varied stresses such as toxins, radiation and inflammatory foods.[144] Typically, endocrine function is compromised initially, meaning that people can't produce enough insulin to store blood sugar, which leads to type 2 diabetes.

Excocrine function can be compromised, too, meaning that not enough enzymes like protease, lipase and amylase are made; enzymes are used to break macronutrients into

143. Rossignol, D.A., et al, Melatonin in Autism Spectrum Disorders, *Curr Clin Pharmacol.* 2013 Sep 20.
144. Sircus, Mark, *Sodium Bicarbonate - Full Medical Review.* International Medical Veritas Association, 2010, Kindle locations 411-412.

component parts. For example, protease breaks protein down into its constituent amino acids.

Children with Sensory Processing Disorder and other neurodevelopmental disorders are typically deficient in pancreatic enzymes that are both necessary for digestion and destroy pathogenic viruses, bacteria and cancer cells.[145]

Testing for Nutritional Deficiencies

Two of the most comprehensive nutritional profiles are both offered by Genova Diagnostics: the CardioION profile and the NutrEval. Both are fairly expensive, and not all doctors order tests from this lab, so check with your practitioner first. Functional-medicine doctors and naturopaths are the two types of practitioners that are most likely to offer these lab tests.

Be careful to read through your child's results, as many doctors typically only look for the "L" (low) or "H" (high) flag next to a level. Your child's levels may be on the cusp of being too low or too high, which is why you need to take the time to scan the results thoroughly. Be sure to request copies of all test results for your own records; no one knows your child better than you do.

Magnesium Deficiency Testing

Both the CardioION and NutrEval profiles test for magnesium. If you don't have access to these tests, ask your doctor for an RBC magnesium profile.

Zinc Deficiency Testing

Here's a fun way to test for a zinc deficiency, which is common in many people, especially those with compromised

145. Horvath, K., et al, Gastrointestinal abnormalities in children with autistic disorder, *J Pediatr.* 1999 Nov;135(5):559-63.

immune systems and those who are picky eaters: do a zinc challenge. It's very easy to do: buy some Zinc Challenge, put a little in a cup, have your child swish it in their mouth, then spit it out. It will taste different depending on their zinc status.

People with a zinc deficiency commonly have either a poor sense or a hyper-sensitive sense of taste and smell, and they won't be able to taste the zinc sulfate monohydrate that's in Zinc Challenge. Those with sufficient zinc will notice that it tastes like old eggs and will want to spit it out immediately. In my experience, most people think it tastes like water. Be sure not to tell anyone ahead of time (especially kids) what kind of tastes to expect!

Both the CardioION and NutrEval profiles test for zinc, and there may be other tests out there that test for it as well that I am not aware of.

Iodine Deficiency Testing

David Brownstein, MD, author of *Iodine: Why You Need It, Why You Can't Live Without It*, recommends taking an iodine-loading test first to see how much is excreted. Labs that perform this test are:

- FFP Lab: www.ffplab.org
- Hakala Labas: www.hakalalabs.com
- Labrix: www.labrix.com

You can also try a rudimentary iodine test at home on your child: Put some Lugol's iodine on his or her skin. It should be there for 24-48 hours. If not, your child is likely deficient.

Neither the CardioION nor NutrEval tests for iodine.

Iron Deficiency Testing

Most doctors have basic labs that test for iron levels. However, if you're having your child tested for this, also have your doctor test for ferritin, which is the storage form of iron.

Vitamin D Deficiency Testing

Your pediatrician should be able to order a vitamin D test; just make sure it's the "25-hydroxy" test. Both the CardioION and NutrEval profiles test for vitamin D levels.

Optimal levels are above 80, despite the fact that 30 to 70 is considered "normal"; a level of 50 or less is insufficient.[146] "Normal" isn't healthy anymore; you want optimal for your child.

Essential Fatty Acids Deficiencies Testing

Both the NutrEval and CardioION test for common fatty acid deficiencies such as DHA, EPA, ALA, GLA and LA, which should be sufficient in determining targeted supplementation for your child. If your practitioner has access to it and you want a more in-depth analysis of more than 40 different fatty acids, the BodyBio profile by Kennedy Krieger at Johns Hopkins is an excellent choice.

Glutathione Deficiency Testing

Although the CardioION does not test for glutathione levels, the NutrEval does.

Stomach Acid Deficiency Testing

The easiest and cheapest way for you to test stomach acid

---

146. Rogers, Sherry, MD, *Total Wellness Newsletter*, March 2014, 4.

levels is for you to do a test at home on your child. Put ¼ teaspoon of baking soda in eight ounces of water. Have your child drink it. If he or she burps within two minutes, there is a sufficient amount of stomach acid for proper digestion.

Methyl Deficiencies Testing

Both the NutrEval and CardioION test for B vitamins, but your pediatrician can order simple blood tests for these, too. You're interested in levels of vitamin B_5, vitamin B_6 and vitamin B_{12} for these purposes. In the case of vitamin B_{12}, a urine test may also be in order because sometimes blood levels of B_{12} look fine, but it's not getting absorbed. If that's the case, most of it would be eliminated through urine. A B_{12} deficiency is called pernicious anemia, and a person with this typically lacks intrinsic factor, a protein made in the stomach.

The test for the MTHFR genetic defect is fairly simple and cheap ($150 from Spectracell Labs), considering that knowing how to circumvent the problem can help you avoid so much pain and sickness in your child's life. The condition is correctable with proper supplementation.

Amino Acid Deficiencies Testing

Both the CardioION and NutrEval test for some amino acids, but not GABA and carnitine. Your pediatrician should be able to order labs for all amino acids with standard lab tests.

Melatonin Deficiency Testing

Genova Diagnostics offers a 24-hour melatonin assay, although testing for tryptophan levels may be a good proxy. Consider that your child may have a melatonin deficiency if, after exhausting all methods listed in the "Optimizing Sleep" section, your child still has trouble falling and staying asleep.

Pancreatic Enzyme Deficiencies Testing

Although the CardioION does not test for pancreatic enzymes levels, the NutrEval does. In addition, Genova's Comprehensive Digestive Stool Analysis tests for this. There may be other available tests out there that your practitioner has access to that I am not aware of.

Hormonal Imbalances

Hormonal imbalances are a commonly overlooked causative factor in children with neurodevelopmental disorders. Children with Sensory Processing Disorder are very likely to have adrenal fatigue because their bodies are always dealing with the stress of incorrect sensory processing. In addition, there's usually a 75-80% overlap between adrenal fatigue and low thyroid function. If your child has one, he or she very likely has the other.

Adrenal Fatigue

Most people wouldn't even consider that their child with Sensory Processing Disorder has adrenal fatigue because of their age, but your child's behavior may be telling you otherwise.

Symptoms of Adrenal Fatigue

Chronic fatigue, sickness, tantrums and irritability are often indicative of adrenal fatigue in a child. You have to remember that a child's actions speak louder than words. Other signs and symptoms of adrenal fatigue are:

- Difficulty getting up in the morning
- Continuing fatigue not relieved by sleep
- Craving for salt or salty foods

- Lethargy (lack of energy)
- Increased effort to do everyday tasks
- Decreased ability to handle stress
- Increased time to recover from illness, injury or trauma
- Symptoms increase if meals are skipped or inadequate
- Decreased stamina
- Blood-sugar swings
- Anxiety

I found a great discussion of these symptoms in the book, *Adrenal Fatigue: The 21st Century Stress Syndrome*, by James L. Wilson. He says that, "Chronic and recurrent bronchitis, pneumonia and other chronic lung and bronchial diseases typically have an adrenal fatigue component. This includes many cases of asthma, influenza and allergies."[147] My older son had constant eczema, which was worse in the winter, and later developed a life-threatening bout of asthma when he was just over four years old in which he was on prednisolone, Xopenex, and a nebulizer.

Causes of Adrenal Fatigue

Unfortunately, your child has been born into a high-stress age! Anything that causes stress, especially if it's chronic, can cause insufficient output from your child's adrenal glands.

Stress

Chronic stress can wear out your child's adrenal glands. Stress can come from toxicity, a nutrient-poor lifestyle, emotional stress, faulty sensory processing, retained reflexes, EMFs and constant sickness as well as just plain old running around too much to activities like soccer practice and baseball games. Your child needs downtime, especially in this day and age of highly structured schedules.

---

147. Wilson, James O., *Adrenal Fatigue: The 21st Century Stress Syndrome.* Petaluma, CA: Smart Publications, 2001, 49.

Passed from Mother to Child

The stress response can be inherited.[148] Mothers who experience stress, especially chronic stress, during pregnancy are much more likely to have a child with an inability to handle stress, whether it's in the form of Sensory Processing Disorder, anxiety, mood swings or irritability. I often wonder if my high-stress Wall Street job was a factor in my older son's more-severe SPD because I was still working when I was pregnant with him.

Toxicity

Toxicity is a constant source of stress in your child's body. Toxicity causes oxidative stress, otherwise known as inflammation. The adrenal glands produce cortisol to counteract inflammation, but constant cortisol production can wear them out. A child with toxin overload is likely to have blood-sugar swings because cortisol is also needed to control blood sugar, and if it's being used for inflammation instead, your child won't have enough cortisol left to manage blood sugar.

Sugar

Sugar, especially an excess of it or if eaten alone, causes adrenal fatigue. Cortisol, made by the adrenal glands, controls blood-sugar swings. Too much sugar can cause excess cortisol production, leading eventually to adrenal fatigue, where your child's adrenals can't make enough cortisol to get him or her through the day with enough energy. Sugar also decreases your child's ability to concentrate. A high-sugar diet leads to a lack

148. Seong, K.H., Inheritance of stress-induced, ATF-2-dependent epigenetic change, *Cell.* 2011 Jun 24;145(7):1049-61.

of attention in children (and adults, too!) as well as an increase in adrenaline.[149]

Nutritional Deficiencies

Minerals feed the adrenal glands and keep it functioning properly. Key minerals for the adrenals are magnesium, zinc, selenium and chromium, although trace minerals are important as well. In our era of high stress and highly processed foods, it's likely that your child's adrenals are starving. Cravings for sweet and/or salty foods are typical in a child with adrenal fatigue.

Faulty Sensory Processing

Constant sensory stress causes surges of adrenaline and cortisol that can create a vicious cycle that ends in the adrenals not being able to produce enough cortisol to deal with the stress.

Retained Reflexes

Children with neurodevelopmental disorders such as Sensory Processing Disorder typically have reflexes that have been retained that should have been integrated when they were babies. These retained reflexes are the result of a damaged nervous system and are part and parcel of your child's sensory issues. I'll discuss them more in the "Understanding Retained Reflexes" chapter, but just know for now that the presence of them causes stress for your child that can result in fatigued adrenal glands.

My older son's adrenal fatigue stressed his body so much that he was constantly getting sick. He would go to preschool

---

149. http://www.yalescientific.org/2010/09/mythbusters-does-sugar-really-make-children-hyper/. Accessed September 2, 2014.

for a week and be out the whole next week because he had gotten sick. This scenario played out for the whole first year of preschool when he was three and got slightly better the next year after he started going to OTs because their work on neuromuscular reeducation, vestibular reeducation, and core strengthening was helping to inhibit some of his retained Moro reflex, the "fight, fright or flight" reflex.

EMFs

Constant exposure to EMFs puts your child's body in a state of constant stress. Wi-Fi systems, cell phones, cell towers, cordless phones, dirty electricity, smart meters, tablet devices and large electrical appliances are the most common causes of EMFs in your child's life. If you live in a city, your child's EMF exposure is much higher. Constant stress of being exposed to EMFs can fatigue the adrenals of your child.

Constant Sickness

The stress of being constantly sick with colds, allergies, asthma and infections places undue energy demands on your child's body. It's likely that a child with these issues also has adrenal fatigue.

Testing for Adrenal Fatigue

You may want to have an Adrenal Stress Profile test performed by your functional-medicine or naturopathic doctor first, but an easy way to check for adrenal fatigue is to go into a dark bathroom and shine a flashlight in your or your child's eyes while looking in the mirror. If the eye dilates rather than stays constricted, this is a good indicator of adrenal fatigue.

Cortisol is made by the adrenal glands. Not only does it control inflammation, but it also controls blood sugar. For that reason, you'll want to get a blood glucose monitor to check your child's fasting and non-fasting blood sugar at home. A few of my clients have discovered that they were either pre-diabetic or flat-out diabetic, so checking yourself at home is a great way to stay on top of this potentially debilitating problem, especially because children with Sensory Processing Disorder are more likely to have blood-sugar problems. Fasting blood sugar should be no higher than 100, although 85 is more optimal, and blood sugar a half hour after eating should be no higher than 140.

Low Thyroid Function

Dr. Raphael Kellman, a holistic endocrinologist in New York City, believes that 70-80% of children with Sensory Processing Disorder, autism, developmental delays, ADHD, PDD-NOS are hypothyroid.[150] I believe hypothyroidism, as well as adrenal fatigue and systemic *Candida* infection, may be the great under-reported factors of Sensory Processing Disorder, as well as the epidemic of other chronic illnesses in both children and adults.

Symptoms of Low Thyroid Function

If your child's thyroid isn't working properly, neither is his or her immune system. The key feature of an under-functioning thyroid is a low body temperature. A body temperature of 97.8° Fahrenheit or below is indicative of an underactive thyroid gland. My older son's temperature was typically in the high 96s, low 97s. When I asked the pediatric nurses about this, they waved it off as if it were no big deal. It is. Other key symptoms of low thyroid function are:

- Fatigue
- Sluggishness
- Poor coordination

---

150. Kellman, Raphael, MD, *The Thyroid-Autism Connection*, AutismOne Conference 2012, www.autismone.orgcontent/thyroid-autism-connection-2

- Increased sensitivity to cold
- Pale, dry skin
- Brittle fingernails and hair
- Depression
- Anxiety
- Scalloped tongue
- Poor digestion
- Low body temperature
- Cold hands and feet
- Adrenal fatigue likely
- High cholesterol
- Thick-tongued speech
- Low stamina
- Low motivation
- Forgetfulness
- Foggy thinking
- Irritability
- Poor immunity; constant sickness
- Low blood pressure
- Drowsiness

In addition, hypothyroidism in children doesn't necessarily mean that they have unexplained weight gain, which is what typically happens to an adult. Indeed, these children may even be poor growers, like my boys. Additional symptoms to look for in children are:

- Hypotonia
- Fine-motor problems
- Repetitive behavior
- Social dysfunction
- Poor growth, resulting in short stature
- Delayed puberty
- Delayed development of permanent teeth
- Cognitive dysfunction
- Attention problems
- Hyperactivity

Causes of Low Thyroid Function

With the constant stress that our children are exposed to today, whether it's from emotional stress, toxic stress, or goitrogenic foods, it's a wonder that most children today don't have underactive thyroids. In addition, gluten sensitivity and nutritional deficiencies are often overlooked as causes for hypothyroidism.

Passed from Mother to Child

A mother that is hypothyroid is more likely to have a child that is hypothyroid. This is typically because the child's mother was hypothyroid when pregnant. This hypothyroid condition affects the way the fetus' brain and central nervous system develop.[151]

Stress

Stress, especially chronic stress, can affect the ability of the thyroid to do its job well. Even happy events like moving to a new house or school can cause stress because what matters is that it's a big-enough change from the way things used to be.

Endocrine Disruptors

As I've shown you, our children's bodies are exposed to an outrageous number of endocrine disruptors these days, even before birth. Toxins such as pesticides, heavy metals, fluoride, chlorine, bromine, flame retardants, PCBs, perchlorate, DDT, BPA, BPS, non-stick coatings, waterproof coatings, parabens, phthalates, plastics, plasticizers, acetone and triclosan have all

---

151. Colborn, Theo, Neurodevelopment and Endocrine Disruption, *Environ Health Perspect.* 2004 Jun;112(9):944-9.

been shown to have a detrimental effect on the thyroid's function.

Inflammation

Having antibodies against the receptors for thyroid-stimulating hormone is a hidden cause of hypothyroidism, despite having "normal" TSH levels and taking thyroid medication.[152] In addition, Kelly Brogan, MD, says that many people with low thyroid have Hashimoto's, an autoimmune disease of the thyroid, and that "as many as 20% of people have circulating antibodies indicative of Hashimoto's thyroiditis."[153]

Goitrogenic Foods

Consumption of goitrogenic foods such as unfermented soy products and raw, cruciferous vegetables can disrupt the function of the thyroid. Examples of unfermented soy products are:

- Tofu
- Soy milk
- Soy protein isolates
- Soy beans
- Edamame
- Soy flour
- Textured vegetable protein

Examples of raw goitrogenic foods are:

---

152. http://drclark.typepad.com/dr_david_clark/2012/11/hidden-cause-9-why-you-still-have-low-thyroid-symptoms.html. Accessed September 14, 2014.
153. http://us7.campaign-archive1.com/?u=12bbf28aa99bdf62c30e5c10c&id=801769f4fb&e=cb96a7625a. Accessed September 14, 2014.

- Kale
- Broccoli
- Cauliflower
- Bok choy
- Cabbage
- Other cruciferous vegetables
- Spinach
- Non-organic strawberries

Gut Dysbiosis

Recent research indicates that gut microbes influence endocrine function. As an example, "animals raised in a germ-free environment show exaggerated responses to psychological stress, which normalizes following mono-colonization by certain bacterial species."[154]

Gluten

Both clinical research and client evidence support the claim that gluten adversely affects thyroid function.[155] Gluten is found in wheat, rye, barley and non-gluten-free oats. As stated earlier, it might not be the gluten that's the problem; it might be what's been done to it, as the pesticide Roundup® (glyphosate) is typically sprayed on wheat crops.

Nutritional Deficiencies

Mineral deficiencies are a common cause of low thyroid function. The most essential minerals for your child's thyroid are iodine, selenium and zinc, with iodine being the most important, says David Brownstein, MD, in *Iodine: Why You*

154. Clarke, G., et al, Minireview: gut microbiota: the neglected endocrine organ, *Mol Endocrinol.* 2014 Aug;28(8):1221-38.
155. Ringvold, H., [Gluten intolerance, hypothyroidism, lactose and fructose malabsorption--a new "syndrome"?], *Tidsskr Nor Laegeforen.* 2006 Sep 7;126(17):2286.

Need It, Why You Can't Live Without It. Your child doesn't have to have a goiter to be iodine deficient; Dr. Brownstein says that 92% of his patients tested low for iodine levels.[156]

Testing for Thyroid Dysfunction

The basal body temperature (BBT) test developed by Dr. Broda Barnes years ago is still a reliable indicator of hypothyroidism. You can test your child at home by sticking a thermometer under the arm for five to 10 minutes, preferably before your child gets out of bed in the morning. If the reading is 97.8° Fahrenheit or lower, your child is likely hypothyroid, and this can warrant further testing.

Most doctors will typically run a test for TSH (thyroid stimulating hormone), but it's a typically unreliable test for diagnosing hypothyroidism. See if your doctor can test your child for T3, T4, free T3, free T4, reverse T3 and thyroid antibodies.

Dr. Kellman says that the typical TSH test misses an underactive thyroid. Instead, he recommends a TRH (thyroid releasing hormone) test, which he says that most doctors used to use until the TSH came into vogue because it's cheaper and faster. However, few doctors now use the TRH test. With the TRH test, TRH, a compound of the hypothalamus controlled by the pituitary, is injected into the patient's bloodstream. Blood is drawn about 30 minutes later to see if the TRH stimulated the pituitary to release a lot of TSH. A normal person's reading is around 10; a person with hypothyroidism has a level above 10.

Inflammation

Inflammation is a root cause of many chronic illnesses such as Sensory Processing Disorder, autism, ADHD, allergies,

---

156. Brownstein, David, MD, ***Iodine:*** *Why You Need It, Why You Can't Live Without It.* West Bloomfield, MI: Medical Alternative Press, 2009, 49.

asthma, eczema, lupus, fibromyalgia, rheumatoid arthritis, autoimmune diseases, heart disease, type 2 diabetes and metabolic syndrome. In neurodevelopmental disorders like Sensory Processing Disorder, autism and ADHD, inflammation also takes the form of neuroinflammation.[157]

Symptoms of Inflammation

Inflammation causes pain, swelling, heat, redness and loss of function. In a child with neuroinflammation, neural processes can go haywire: senses aren't processed correctly, executive functions aren't executed properly and your child's ability for reasoning and interacting socially are lowered.

Causes of Inflammation

If you've read this far in the book, you can probably guess what the causes of inflammation are: maternal inheritance, toxicity, sugar/processed foods, nutritional deficiencies, stress and EMFs. What you may not have realized is that certain other foods, especially vegetable oils and trans fats, are also highly inflammatory.

Passed from Mother to Child

A history of autoimmune disease in the family is a big risk factor for having a child with Sensory Processing Disorder, autism, ADHD, allergies, asthma or autoimmune. That's because mom's inflammation during pregnancy gets passed on to her baby. In a recent research study, inflammation was measured by the amount of C-reactive protein (CRP) in a pregnant woman's blood. Results were striking: Pregnant women with CRP in the top 20th percentile have a 43% increased risk of having a child with autism. Pregnant women

157. Theoharides TC, et al, Focal brain inflammation and autism, *J Neuroinflammation.* 2013 Apr 9;10:46.

whose CRP is in the top 10th percentile have a whopping 80% higher risk of having an autistic child.[158] Just because this study looked at only autistic children, don't think it doesn't apply to your SPD child; it does. Additional research now shows that prenatal stress has an impact on a child's health and mental health.[159]

Toxicity

Toxins cause inflammation in your child's body. Heavy metals are well known for their ability to cause inflammation. In addition, endocrine disruptors that contribute to a mother's and baby's hypothyroidism also cause inflammation.[160]

Sugar and Processed Foods

Sugar causes inflammation. Sugary foods cause an increase of inflammatory cytokines. An overproduction or inappropriate production of certain cytokines by the body can result in diseases like heart disease, cancer and autoimmune diseases.[161]

High-Fructose Corn Syrup

Scientists now believe that high-fructose corn syrup plays

---

158. Brown, A.S. et al, Elevated maternal C-reactive protein and autism in a national birth cohort. *Molecular Psychiatry*, 2013; DOI: 10.1038/mp.2012.197
159. Glover, V., Annual Research Review: Prenatal stress and the origins of psychopathology: an evolutionary perspective, *J Child Psychol Psychiatry.* 2011 Apr;52(4):356-67.
160. Sajdel-Sulkowska, Elizabeth M., "Environmentally Induced Oxidative Stress and Disruption of Brain Thyroid Hormone Homeostasis in Autism Spectrum Disorders", *Autism - A Neurodevelopmental Journey from Genes to Behaviour,* Edited by Valsamma Eapen, InTech, 2011.
161. http://www.health.harvard.edu/fhg/updates/What-you-eat-can-fuel-or-cool-inflammation-a-key-driver-of-heart-disease-diabetes-and-other-chronic-conditions.shtml. Accessed September 1, 2014.

a unique and causal role in the etiology of diabetes. One of the reasons is that it causes mitochondrial oxidative stress.[162]

Vegetable Oils

Vegetable oils are processed at high heats, which immediately makes them inflammatory. To add insult to injury, they are then deodorized and bleached to remove the smell of their rancidity.

Canola oil has been found to deplete vitamin E… an antioxidant.[163] So by eating canola oil, your child is actually lowering levels of antioxidants rather than increasing them, like the label on the canola oil bottle promises. That's a real problem because 95% of wealthy kids under the age of five are deficient in vitamin E. If wealthy kids are deficient and they have access to potentially healthier foods, then what about the rest of the population?

Canola also increases the rigidity of cell membranes, which is a real concern for those with autism, SPD and ADHD, who have often been found to have mitochondrial dysfunction.

Canola oil also contains erucic acid, a neurotoxin, which is why it's not allowed in baby formula. If it's not allowed in formula, why is it OK for the rest of us to eat? I'm picking on canola the most because it's so often touted as having the most health benefits, when research is showing that its real impact is quite the opposite.

One of my pet peeves is going to Whole Foods and finding a lot of their prepared foods in the hot bar and deli section contain canola oil, but, hey, at least they list it on the ingredient label. Still, I think most people assume that if it's sold in Whole Foods, it must be healthy, but even there you can't let your guard down.

Canola oil and other vegetable oils are usually found in

---

162. Johnson, R.J., Sugar, uric acid, and the etiology of diabetes and obesity, *Diabetes*. 2013 Oct;62(10):3307-15.

163. Sauer, FD, et al, Additional vitamin E required in milk replacer diets that contain canola oil, *Nutr Res* 17; 2:259-69, 1997

processed foods, too: chips, cookies, crackers, bread, salad dressings, mayonnaise and more. It's really hard to find processed foods that don't contain them!

What's really disheartening is that restaurants that brag about not using trans fats in their foods are now using vegetable oils instead. Did you know that McDonald's used to cook their fries in lard or tallow up until 1990?

Two great sources to educate yourself about the dangers of eating vegetable oils are the Weston A. Price Foundation's "The Oiling of America" article[164] and Udo Erasmus' book, *Fats That Heal, Fats That Kill.*

Trans Fats

Canola is the biggest deceiver of them all. You see, we're all told that canola has a higher level of omega-3 oils. We think, "Great! Omega-3 oils lower inflammation." Not so fast. With all of the processing done to it, canola oil on the shelf contains as much as 40% trans fatty acids, even more than soybean oil.[165]

Dr. Sherry Rogers, one of my favorite biomedical doctors, says that she started investigating canola oil because even though her patients weren't knowingly eating trans fatty acids, their CardioION results showed progressively higher levels of them.

Canola isn't the only source of trans fats. They're found in anything with "partially hydrogenated" or "hydrogenated" on the label. And don't be fooled by "trans fat free" on the label because manufacturers are lowering portion sizes so that trans fat levels are less than 0.5g per serving. If that's the case, they are allowed to round the level down to zero and make that

---

164. http://www.westonaprice.org/health-topics/the-oiling-of-america/. Accessed September 14, 2014.

165. Rogers, Sherry. The Canola Con… It's Worse Than the Soy Ploy, *Dr. Sherry Rogers' Total Wellness*, January 2010, 3.

claim. Harvard Medical School has said "There is no safe level of trans fats".[166]

Even if cookies, crackers, chips, breads, cakes and whatever processed foods don't list "partially hydrogenated" or "hydrogenated" on the label, foods made with vegetable oils, especially canola and soy, will have trans fats in them, even though the label says "trans fat free." In addition, never allow your child to eat margarine or any kind of shelf-stable vegetable oil, even if it makes the claim that it's healthy. It's not.

Nutritional Deficiencies

Deficiencies of antioxidants such as vitamin A, vitamin C and vitamin E in the diet as well as essential fatty acid deficiencies can leave your SPD child in an inflamed state. In addition, most SPD children, as mentioned, also have a glutathione deficiency.

Stress

Stress causes inflammation, and I think a lot of people underestimate the impact that emotional stress has on health. Stressful emotions like anger, frustration and hopelessness can cause immune dysregulation and inflammation.

EMFs

Exposure to EMFs such as those from cell phones, cordless phones, Wi-Fi, plasma TVs and more can put the body into a state of "fight or flight," even when your child is sleeping.[167] A body under constant stress is a body with

---

166. http://www.health.harvard.edu/fhg/updates/Truth-about-fats.shtml. Accessed September 14, 2014.
167. Nazıroğlu M, et al, Recent reports of Wi-Fi and mobile phone-induced radiation on oxidative stress and reproductive signaling pathways in females

constant inflammation and one that can't properly detoxify. EMFs, including those known as "dirty electricity," also make fungi (mold, yeast, etc.) more virulent, and this was known at least as far back as 1980.[168]

Testing for Inflammation

Consider getting CRP (C-reactive protein) and homocysteine tests from your doctor to check your child for inflammation. These are common tests available from most doctors.

Other Factors

In addition to the usual suspects of toxicity, gut dysbiosis, immune dysregulation, nutritional deficiencies and inflammation, there may be other factors at play in causing your child's Sensory Processing Disorder. Ultrasounds, traumatic birth experiences, back sleeping, vertebral subluxation and being a boy are also potential risk factors.

Ultrasounds

Medical research confirms that "fetal exposure to diagnostic ultrasound applied in utero can alter typical social behaviors in young mice that may be relevant for autism."[169] Jennifer Margulis, PhD, explains why in great detail in her book, *The Business of Baby: What Doctors Don't Tell You, What Corporations Try to Sell You, and How to Put Your Pregnancy, Childbirth, and Baby Before Their Bottom Line.*

---

and males, *J Membr Biol.* 2013 Dec;246(12):869-75.
168. Mezykowski T, Response of Aspergillus nidulans and Physarum polycephalum to microwave irradiation, *J Microw Power.* 1980 Jun;15(2):75-80.
169. McClintic, A.M., Mice exposed to diagnostic ultrasound in utero are less social and more active in social situations relative to controls, *Autism Res.* 2014 Jun;7(3):295-304.

Traumatic Birth Experience

Birth trauma is another risk factor for a child developing a neurodevelopmental disorder or developmental delay, likely due to deprivation of oxygen. As an example, babies deprived of oxygen before birth are far more likely to have ADHD later in life. Babies that experienced birth trauma or fetal distress such as birth asphyxia, neonatal respiratory distress syndrome and preeclampsia are 16% more likely to have ADHD.[170]

My older son had a very traumatic birth experience. I was in labor for several hours when all of a sudden the nursing team couldn't find his heartbeat. At this point, they broke my water so they could insert a monitor to listen to it. They found it, but when they broke the water, my son went into fetal distress, and I was wheeled into the surgery room for an emergency C-section.

My doctor, who had not yet shown up, was finally contacted, and she halted the surgery. I was then told to relax (yeah, right) for several hours so the anesthetic they had given me for emergency surgery could wear off. Pitocin was then administered to restart labor, and when my son finally emerged, he had meconium in his lungs, which then had to be immediately suctioned. His APGAR score was 5/9.

Boys

Just being a boy raises the risk of having a chronic health condition like autism, ADHD or SPD. The number of autistic boys outweighs the number of autistic girls by a ratio of about four to one. Current research believes that is due to the expression of estrogen receptor beta, which plays a role in anxiety, depression, memory, learning, behavior and locomotion. This receptor enables estrogen's brain protection

---

170. Getahun, D., et al, In utero exposure to ischemic-hypoxic conditions and attention-deficit/hyperactivity disorder, *Pediatrics.* 2013 Jan;131(1):e53-61.

and is significantly decreased in the brains of autistic children.[171]

Back Sleeping

Putting a baby to sleep on their back is like having their nervous system "upside down", Patricia Lemer often says. Babies who sleep on their backs don't develop as they should: their core, neck, wrist and hand muscles are often weak because they're not using those muscles to push themselves up and over, and this can lead to the retention of primitive reflexes, which I'll go over later in the book. An example of the far-reaching effects of this practice can be seen in today's kindergarteners who often lack the fine motor skills necessary for proper handwriting. Carrying a baby in a bucket seat or in a stroller, and putting a baby in a bouncy seat or in an upright walker before they're walking are other ways that cause a baby not to develop gross and fine motor skills that are so necessary for proper nervous-system integration.

Vertebral Subluxation

The multitudes of neurodevelopmental toxins that I've described as well as emotional and birth trauma can create what a chiropractor would call "vertebral subluxation", which is interference in the nervous system's communication. Vertebral subluxation can speed up or slow down the rate at which nervous-system messages travel. The result is that a child's brain cannot properly communicate with the rest of the body and vice versa.

Epigenetics

I believe there is far too much time, money and attention paid to researching genetic origins of diseases and to

171. Crider, A., et al, Dysregulation of estrogen receptor beta (ERβ), aromatase (CYP19A1), and ER co-activators in the middle frontal gyrus of autism spectrum disorder subjects. *Molecular Autism*, 2014; 5 (1): 46

developing pharmaceuticals that mask symptoms. Why are we spending millions of dollars trying to find a cure for autism or cancer, for example, and not looking at what can be done to prevent it or what causes it?

- Toxins that increase the risk
- Foods that can reduce the risk
- Foods that can increase the risk
- Supplements that can decrease the risk
- Stress and inflammation that increase the risk

Why? Because there's no money in prevention. OK, maybe a little, but it's nothing in comparison to the money that is generated by a drug that provides a temporary benefit and simply masks a symptom without getting to the root cause.

As Robyn O'Brien said in *The Unhealthy Truth: One Mother's Shocking Investigation into the Dangers of America's Food Supply– and What Every Family Can Do to Protect Itself*: "Our commercialized health-care system turns us into little profit centers for the drug industry and the medical establishment, so there's no similar incentive to prevent health problems."[172] In other words, your child is worth more as a sick person because they need drugs and medical services to treat their condition, which costs money, certainly far more money than it would have cost them to eat healthy food, correct nutritional deficiencies and detoxify.

Bruce Lipton, author of *The Biology of Belief*, believes that only 3-5% of disease is genetic; the rest is epigenetic. The basic premise is "genetics loads the gun, environment pulls the trigger," Yes, your child may carry a certain gene, which means he or she is more likely to have Sensory Processing Disorder, but what your child eats and drinks, what they put on their skin, what toxins they're born with and the toxins they're exposed to, how they deal with stress, how healthy their gut flora is, and whether or not they take pharmaceuticals, hormones or over-the-counter drugs is far more important.

---

172. O'Brien, Robyn, *The Unhealthy Truth: One Mother's Shocking Investigation into the Dangers of America's Food Supply – and What Every Family Can Do to Protect Itself*. New York, NY: Broadway Books, 2009, 177.

The really great thing is that environmental and nutritional factors are likely to moderate genetic risk, so what your child eats and supplements with can make a huge difference. And, as a parent, it's in your control to make a difference!

FINDING HELP: OUR STORY

It can be difficult to find help if you don't know what you're dealing with. For my older son, I had a litany of signs for 3 ½ years that told me something was wrong, despite reassurances to the contrary of his doctors. I didn't know whom to turn to for help. Help! A few months after my older son started preschool, his teachers alerted me that he cried and cried all the time one day while he was at school. It was a very dark and rainy day, and apparently my son thought that it was nighttime and that I had neglected to pick him up, which wasn't the case. Finally, I had something more definitive and concrete to go on.

I wanted to rule out any kind of physical problem, so I took him to the pediatrician. It turned out that my son had an ear infection. Still, I thought his reaction was excessive, and I told her so and reminded her of some of the other things I thought were unusual, such as the fact that he didn't walk until he was 20 months old. Although she couldn't come up with a diagnosis, she referred me to a psychiatric nurse practitioner that specializes in children's behavioral problems, who then referred me to an occupational therapist (OT).

Before we began working with the OT, she had me fill out a sensory profile and a sensory questionnaire. Here are some of my comments from the profile and questionnaire:

- Is "very good at hiding pain; past two ear infections were within the past four months, and he never complained about the pain."
- Can be "stubborn or uncooperative when asked to do something physically."
- "Intent on controlling/manipulating to keep environment predictable: a little dictator."
- "Often very inactive, unmoving or lethargic."
- "Seems to require too much sleep at odd times. Took two naps a day up until 18 months of age; can still take three-hour naps at times."
- "Difficulty walking up/down flights of stairs: doesn't alternate feet."
- "Maintains rigid and repetitive patterns or 'rules'; extremely long, involved and rigid bedtime routine."
- "Avoids age-appropriate participation in group gross-motor activities."
- "Cannot lift heavy objects, avoids heavy work."
- "Resists new physical challenges; says 'I can't' without attempting. Even says 'I can't' to things he can do. Is he lazy or tired? We don't know."
- "Seems weaker or tires more easily than peers."
- "Swimming (group) class at two years of age was a disaster. He would not pay attention to the instructor because he was too distracted by lights and surroundings. He was so frustrated after a few weeks of going to class that he wiped down half the kitchen one day after class. We never went back."
- "Gym class was a disaster because he would lie on the floor and suck his fingers for most of the class."

So guess which one of these comments gave the biggest clue as to what we were dealing with. Give up? It was "cannot lift heavy objects; avoids heavy work." The story behind this comment was that my two sons were playing with a heavy glass blender carafe one day on the kitchen floor. My younger son, who is 21 months younger and about a year and a half old at the time, could lift it while my older one could not, despite how hard he tried.

From my answers, I began to see that my son had pretty severe sensory issues. I began to read everything I could about SPD. I found *The Out-of-Sync Child: Recognizing and Coping with Sensory Processing Disorder* by Carol Kranowitz and Lucy Jane Miller to be an extremely helpful resource. Now at last I began to understand what we were dealing with and that we weren't alone. Finally. Also, the reason that no doctor was able to help is that SPD is not an official diagnosis recognized by the DSM (*Diagnostic and Statistical Manual of Mental Disorders,* which is a reference book for mental health professionals that lists categories of mental disorders and the criteria for diagnosing them), such as autism or ADHD. From a doctor's point of view: no diagnosis, no treatment. Which is why it took so long to get any help.

The good news is that now we finally had an answer. If you know what you're dealing with, then you can get help in treating it.

Catching Problems as Early as Possible

It is my understanding that the earlier the intervention occurs, the better, as children's brains are constantly growing and rewiring themselves. Intervention causes the brain to rewire itself so that the brain properly processes signals from the nervous system. My older son's intervention began when he was 3 ½ years old. That's 3 ½ years of valuable time wasted when the brain is growing and developing at a phenomenal rate. That's why most states have some kind of birth-to-three program because if you can catch developmental delays before a child turns three, the child might not miss out on critical brain-development times. For example, if a child has a speech delay that is not addressed by the time the child is around three or even earlier, then the part of the brain that deals with language might not grow properly and some language function may be permanently lost.

In addition, I believe the younger the child is, the faster he or she can recover. The son of a client of mine, an MD, regressed into autism at the age of six months after the DTaP shot. After working with me and learning about the things I'm teaching you in this book, her son lost his diagnosis at 16 months!

If you were to meet my older son today, you would have no clue that this is the same child I've discussed here. He is happy; he's social; he's even extremely outgoing! Who knew that this was the child that was really hiding inside this damaged body?

Being Scared in His Own Body

My older son began seeing an occupational therapist when he was 3 ½ years old. Before his first visit, she had me fill out two questionnaires: a sensory profile caregiver questionnaire and a foundational listening skills assessment sensory checklist. The answers I gave provided a foundation for her to plan sessions with my son. She noted that my primary reasons for seeking her services were my son's muscle weakness, decreased ability to play with others in a physical manner, and general anxiety.

Caregiver Questionnaire

From the caregiver questionnaire, the OT concluded that my son had probable differences (scores between one and two standard deviations below the mean) in auditory, visual, vestibular and multi-sensory processing. She noted that he had a definite difference (more than two standard deviations below the mean) in oral sensory processing. I believe if I had pushed hard enough, he could've easily qualified for a PDD-NOS (pervasive developmental delay, not otherwise specified) diagnosis.

She evaluated his modulation, which "reflects the child's regulation of neural messages through facilitation or inhibition of various types of responses." My son displayed a probable difference in modulation related to body position and movement and definite differences in sensory processing related to endurance/tone and in sensory input affecting emotional responses.

He showed a probable difference in inattention/distractibility and definite differences in being emotionally reactive (remember all that crying?), low endurance/tone, oral sensitivity, sensory sensitivity and in being sedentary. He also exhibited definite differences in his emotional/social responses and in his behavioral outcome of sensory processing.

Foundational Listening Skills Assessment Sensory Checklist

From the foundational listening skills assessment sensory checklist, she assessed each of his processing systems. Although my son scored in the typical performance range for tactile processing, he showed some areas of concern such as "avoids wearing shoes, prefers to be barefoot and doesn't seem to notice when hands and face are messy" and "is very good at hiding pain." The OT stated that my son appeared to be hypersensitive to sound in reference to him frequently responding "negatively to unexpected loud noises" and to when he stopped what he was doing in her office to acknowledge sounds he heard from outside.

The most important takeaway I got from the sensory checklist was my understanding of my son's scoring a probable difference in vestibular processing, which is responsible for balance and the sense of movement; it is located in both inner ears. I believe this to be the crux of the matter. The OT stated that "the vestibular system is a primary organizer of sensory input in the central nervous system and integrates this information for all of the other sensory systems. It tells us where our head is in space and how fast we are moving. It also has a strong influence on the body's muscle tone and strength as well as helping to maintain a calm, alert state." Aha! Now it was all starting to make sense.

She noted that my son's balance was below normal limits and that he "appeared fearful of movement as witnessed on the swings and tended to keep his head in an upright position." This is why he avoided playground equipment and spent most of his time in sedentary play. She told me that he had "gravitational insecurity" because he didn't understand where his body was in space; he didn't have a reference point because his internal gyroscope was out of balance. Now I understood why he got car sick so often. She also said that because of being so overwhelmed at all these stimuli that were coming at him and not being able to process them that he was scared to be in his own body. How sad!

Vestibular and Proprioceptive Senses

Because his vestibular system was out of balance, so was his proprioceptive sense, otherwise known as "position sense" or "muscle sense." It "gives information about the position of the body without using the eyes and about how much force or pressure is needed to exert to complete a task," such as throwing a ball. The OT noted that my son moved in a "guarded" manner, suggesting that he "moved his body in a calculated manner to protect him from movements that didn't feel safe." This is why he felt like a little limp Raggedy Andy doll when I picked him up; his proprioceptive sense wasn't working correctly because his vestibular system wasn't working correctly.

The OT explained that my son's multi-sensory processing wasn't working correctly, either. He easily became overwhelmed at too much sensory information such as lights and noises and would shut down. She wrote that "when children feel out of control of their bodies with multi-sensory input, they may react to everyday challenges with increased emotional responses." That described my son to a T.

We agreed that she would evaluate him for six sessions and then she would write an evaluation. During these sessions, she tested his abilities such as gross motor coordination: Could he jump two inches off the floor? Could he walk heel-to-toe? Could he hop on one foot one time? These were things he should've been able to do by the age of three, but he still couldn't. She also tested his fine motor coordination and noted that he used an immature grasp and was unable to draw a cross or a square, although he could draw horizontal and vertical lines and a circle.

She evaluated his physical status and noted that he had average to low muscle tone and weak upper and lower extremities. He was unable to hold the "superman" position where your child lies on his or her tummy and lifts both arms and legs up off the floor and was able to make himself into a ball for only a few seconds.

We began seeing immediate results with the OT, even during the six-week evaluation period. Finally! The exercises that she would have my son do, such as swinging on different therapy swings, climbing through tunnels, balancing on one foot, and walking heel-to-toe in a straight line worked on his balance and core strength and gave him strength and confidence very quickly.

She also gave him exercises to do every day at home such as doing a "superman," making himself into a ball and holding the position, rolling like a log, and standing like a statue with his eyes open and closed. She explained that any way that we could get him to move his head in other than a typical position would send information to his vestibular system by making all the fluid and hairs in his inner ears move around and would work to correct his gravitational insecurity.

Within a few weeks of therapy, one day a week, my son became happier and less fearful. He also started tackling us as if he were a football player! He had never been so physical with us before, and it made me so happy to see him acting like a typical kid his age. His teachers at preschool noticed a change, too: they couldn't believe he was the same little boy. He had become much more outgoing and was now the same chatterbox there that he was at home. He loved show-and-tell now and was eager to tell his stories to his classmates. When he started preschool, he engaged in parallel play, and you couldn't get him out of the sand box. By the end of the school year, he had had three months of occupational therapy, and he had moved up to associative play. He even began playing on some of the playground equipment and going on swings and slides! I had been trying to get him to do that since he was a little baby, but he had always cried and refused to do it.

Prior to having OT, my son would always prefer to be with adults, probably because we were more sedentary and predictable than little kids. After receiving OT, his increased confidence allowed him to begin making friendships with children his age. His OT and I talked about the ultimate goal of working with her was for him to make friends. I wasn't expecting my son to become a world-class athlete; I simply wanted him to feel more comfortable with being in his body so that he could make friends. I didn't want to doom him to a life of being socially isolated. This was a tough, but necessary, choice for us because my husband had been recently laid off from his job. Insurance did not cover the OT sessions, and they weren't cheap, but I became convinced after seeing such immediate results that they were well worth it. It was important to correct his imbalances while his brain and nervous system were still growing and developing; trying to correct them at a later age wouldn't have as much of an impact.

The OT said that it was much easier to work with a child like him because he was a sensory avoider; it was like getting him to come out of a box. It was much harder to work with sensory seekers because it was like trying to stuff them back into a box.

My son worked with the OT for six months, at which time she dismissed him for having "strong muscles." I can't say enough good things about her and how much she helped my son. She recommended that he keep up his level of physical activity and said that she liked tae kwon do because of crossing the midline, which helps improve coordination. She also recommended an aquatic OT to help with his swimming.

UNDERSTANDING RETAINED REFLEXES

Many of these toxins that I've described cause neurodevelopmental damage; heavy metals and endocrine disruptors are the usual culprits. Because mom is loaded with these toxins when she's pregnant, it affects the way the baby's brain and nervous system are develops.

What Is a Retained Reflex?

One of the main ways that these neurodevelopmental toxins inflict their damage is by causing a child to retain primitive reflexes that should not have been retained after a certain age. For example, the rooting reflex is a basic reflex babies have that causes them to turn their head to the side in preparation for breastfeeding when that cheek or side of their mouth is touched. If it's not inhibited at round four months of age as nature intended, then it can later to lead to hypersensitivity around the mouth or speech problems.

Retained reflexes are common in children with neurodevelopmental disorders such as autism, PDD-NOS,

ADD/ADHD, Sensory Processing Disorder and learning disabilities.

Evaluation for Retained Reflexes

Not all OTs know about retained reflexes or how to integrate them. Sensory integration therapy isn't necessarily the same as reflex integration. If you're having trouble finding someone in your area that can evaluate your child, I'm going to point you to two books that have some simple tests you can perform on your child at home:

- *Reflexes, Learning and Behavior: A Window into the Child's Mind*, Sally Goddard
- *Ready Bodies, Learning Mind - A Key to Academic Success*, Athena Oden

In any case, if you have a child with a neurodevelopmental disorder, it's almost a given that they have some retained reflexes.

My older son with Sensory Processing Disorder benefited greatly from going to a land-based occupational therapist for six months. I asked her what we should do about him learning to swim, given that he had such a bad experience with it when he was two years old. He had been so overwhelmed by the lights, sounds, the way the water felt, and his gravitational insecurity in the water one day after class he came home and wiped down half the kitchen to relieve his stress. That's a pretty strong reaction from a toddler!

The land-based OT recommended an aquatic OT, whom we began using initially in private sessions after his dismissal from the land-based OT. From their website (www.angelfishtherapy.com): "Aquatic therapy takes place in the water, which is a combination of OT and PT (physical therapy), muscle strengthening, coordination, motor planning, endurance, body awareness and sensory integration."

She (the aquatic OT) didn't give a formal, written evaluation, but, after working with my son a few times, said that he had a couple of retained reflexes that were interfering with his ability to swim. She explained that, as part of typical development, babies naturally inhibit these reflexes, but damage to the central nervous system can cause these reflexes to fail to be inhibited.

Retained Moro Reflex

The aquatic OT said that my son had a retained Moro reflex, the one in which a baby reacts involuntarily to a threat by clinging to its mother. It is also known as the "fight, fright or flight" response and can be caused by neurodevelopmental toxins as well as birth trauma, which is what my older son experienced. To this day, it's not clear why the delivery team couldn't find his heartbeat or why he went into fetal distress, but, for whatever reason, the team discovered that he had released meconium during labor. Upon delivery, the sticky meconium in his lungs prohibited him from breathing, and his lungs had to be suctioned. His one-minute APGAR score was 5, which is a fairly low reading. Maybe this trauma had caused him to retain his Moro reflex.

A retained Moro reflex explained why he had so much anxiety and would cry all the time about everything. His "fight or flight" response couldn't shut off, so there was an almost constant release of adrenaline and cortisol because he felt so out of control and overwhelmed. Poor baby! Now I really felt guilty for getting upset with him those times when his constant crying got to me; it really *wasn't* something he could control!

Sally Goddard writes in *Reflexes, Learning and Behavior: A Window into the Child's Mind* that a child with a retained Moro reflex may have "continued hypersensitivity in one or several sensory channels, causing him to over-react to certain stimuli".[176] This explains why sudden or intense sensory changes upset these children. Some children cope, as mine did, by withdrawing and avoiding sensory changes as much as

176. Goddard, Sally. *Reflexes, Learning and Behavior: A Window into the Child's Mind.* Eugene, OR: Fern Ridge Press, 2005, 6.

possible, while some cope by becoming overactive and aggressive.

Long-Lasting Effects of Retained Moro Reflex

A retained Moro reflex has long-lasting effects on a child, perhaps for life. As I've written, it can profoundly affect a child's ability to make social connections, but it can also create long-term stress and anxiety. What's interesting is that a child who has allergies or asthma may see these conditions disappear or lessen after working on integrating the Moro reflex because the level of stress is lowered.

Other long-term problems that can be caused by a retained Moro reflex are:

- Motion sickness
- Poor balance
- Poor coordination
- Vision problems
- Auditory problems
- Allergies
- Asthma
- Eczema
- Poor stamina
- Difficulty transitioning
- Adrenal fatigue
- Hypoglycemia
- Anxiety
- Mood swings
- Hyperactivity followed by fatigue
- Low self esteem
- Insecurity
- Controlling behavior

Now I knew why grocery shopping with him at a large, echoey, brightly lit grocery store stressed my son out so much!

Retained Symmetric Tonic Neck Reflex (STNR)

The aquatic OT said my son also had a retained symmetric tonic neck reflex (STNR), which should emerge between six and nine months of age and is typically inhibited by nine to 11 months of age. The STNR separates the body's movements from the top half to the bottom half. It's used to help a baby push off the floor to learn cross crawling. If it's integrated, a baby will uncouple the head's movement from the movement of the arms and legs.

Sounds like just a minor point, but it's not. Many kids, like my son, with a retained STNR never cross-crawled or did so for just a short period of time. My son slithered backwards for a couple of months when he first started to move, then he army crawled from eight to 19 months. He cross-crawled for a few weeks and only began to walk at 20 months, which is REALLY late.

A retained STNR can lead to:

- Poor, hunched posture, especially when writing
- Headaches from muscle tension in the neck
- Difficulty writing and reading
- Difficulty sitting still
- "W" sitting
- Difficulty copying from blackboard
- Vision disorders
- Difficulty staying focused
- Clumsiness
- Poor hand-eye coordination
- Difficulty learning to swim, or unsynchronized movements when swimming above the water. (Often children with a retained STNR swim better under the water where the effect of gravity is reduced and the weight of the water keeps the body level.)
- Hypotonia
- Poor upper and lower body integration

Importance of Cross-Crawling

Cross-crawling helps wire the brain's visual processing, which in turn affects learning ability. Think about it: A cross-crawling baby who can bend his neck to look down at the floor then up at his mom mimics the same motion that a child in school does who bends his neck to look at his schoolwork then up to the blackboard.

Cross-crawling, also called "creeping" in some places, coordinates the visual sense, vestibular sense and proprioceptive sense and thus helps a baby develop a sense of balance as well as depth perception. You can see how critical the inhibition of this reflex through cross-crawling is to the child's future learning ability!

Teachers: How many "ADD" or "ADHD" kids that you see in your classroom have poor posture and lack the ability to sit up straight and focus? Could it be they have a retained STNR? Imagine how many children could be taken off of Ritalin if they received proper OT at the proper age of development!

Retained STNR Causes Swimming Difficulty

Because my son had a retained STNR, swimming was difficult for him because kids (and it seems to be mostly boys) with it can't uncouple their head movements from the rest of their bodies, so they swim with their heads back and can't put them down into the water without the back half of their bodies falling down.

Now imagine this reflex being retained in an older child: swimming is almost impossible because the top and bottom halves of the body can't successfully coordinate, while any kind of sport, especially ball games, is a disaster because the child can't coordinate head and eye movements. This child is typically clumsy.

Other Retained Reflexes

There are other retained reflexes that my sons didn't have: palmar reflex, assymetrical tonic reflex, rooting reflex, spinal galant, and tonic labyrinth reflex. Symptoms of these can range from fidgeting, bedwetting, poor concentration, speech difficulties, poor manual dexterity, difficulty crossing the midline, poor balance and poor organization skills. If your child has any of these symptoms, it's worth getting an evaluation from an OT that does primitive reflex integration.

REDUCING STRESS: THE KEY TO RECOVERY

Toxins that children are born with and exposed to, especially heavy metals and endocrine disruptors, can cause neurodevelopmental damage that lead to the development of Sensory Processing Disorder and developmental delays, as well as other neurodevelopmental disorders like autism, ADHD and dyslexia. In addition, research shows that a mother can pass on her stress response that she had during pregnancy to her fetus[1].

Because these toxins and inherited stress response cause undue stress to a child's developing brain and body, the key to recovering your child from these disorders is controlling his or her stress level.

Many of these children have a retained Moro reflex, which causes a constant state of "fight or flight". Because of this, these children experience ongoing, chronic releases of

1. Seong, Ki-Hyeon , et al, Inheritance of Stress-Induced, ATF-2-Dependent Epigenetic Change. *Cell*, 2011; 145 (7): 1049-1061 DOI: 10.1016/j.cell.2011.05.029

adrenaline and cortisol, wearing out their adrenals and immune system. Anyone in this state experiences high amounts of inflammation, which is a key underlying factor in any chronic disease or disorder. However, it's worse in a child with a neurodevelopmental disorder because he or she has chronic neuroinflammation.

A person with high levels of inflammation is more prone to developing food sensitivities, intolerances and allergies, environmental sensitivities and asthma. Thus, lowering stress lowers inflammation and calms the body's response to potential allergens.

Alleviating Anxiety

Clinginess, temper tantrums, constant crying, controlling behavior and difficulty transitioning are all symptoms of an anxious child. This kind of child doesn't respond to reason or logic because, think about it: If you're anxious, you're fearful, and when was the last time you made a great logic-based decision when you were in that kind of state? Instead, it's time to take a look at nutritional deficiencies and a change in the environment, both of which can affect a child's ability to handle stress.

Anxiety and stress cause inflammation in the body[2], so our goal here is to reduce the anxiety, stress and inflammation in your child. Doing so can alleviate some of the symptoms of Sensory Processing Disorder, and I recommend making diet and lifestyle changes first to reduce your child's level of stress.

Optimizing Sleep

Children with neurodevelopmental disorders such as autism, ADHD and Sensory Processing Disorder are

---

2. Maes, M., et al, The effects of psychological stress on humans: increased production of pro-inflammatory cytokines and a Th1-like response in stress-induced anxiety, *Cytokine*. 1998 Apr;10(4):313-8.

notoriously bad sleepers.[3] They have trouble falling asleep and staying asleep. You may hear a noise in the middle of the night and go to your child's room only to discover they are wide awake.

Lack of sleep can cause anxiety in anyone, but especially in a child with a neurodevelopmental disorder because they are typically deficient in many of the nutrients that aid sleep such as glycine, GABA, magnesium and melatonin. I always say that sleep deprivation is a form of torture, and I can say for myself that I am really out of it if I don't get enough sleep!

Glycine and GABA are both amino acids as well as neurotransmitters, and deficiencies of them can cause anxiety and agitation that make it difficult for your child to sleep. One of the best sources of glycine is the gelatin found in home-made bone broth, which is rich in minerals that feed the adrenals and thyroid. Lowering stress for your child reduces the use of critical minerals for counteracting the effects of stress and reserves them for core functions such as sleep.

These children are typically stressed and anxious, and stress uses up an enormous amount of magnesium, a key mineral for both the adrenals and the thyroid. Magnesium also calms the central nervous system, so a child deficient in it will likely have trouble falling asleep. Sugar and processed foods also use up outsized amounts of magnesium for their processing by the body, so lowering the amount of these foods or eliminating them in your child's diet can help your child's ability to sleep.

Children with neurodevelopmental disorders are particularly deficient in melatonin,[4] likely because they are deficient in the amino acid tryptophan, which is the precursor to melatonin; a deficiency in this amino acid could be due to low stomach acid and/or gut dysbiosis. Melatonin is not only a hormone, but it's also an antioxidant. Antioxidants put out

---

3. Krakowiak, P., et al, Sleep problems in children with autism spectrum disorders, developmental delays, and typical development: a population-based study, *J Sleep Res.* 2008 Jun;17(2):197-206.
4. Rossignol, D.A., Melatonin in Autism Spectrum Disorders, *Curr Clin Pharmacol.* 2013 Sep 20.

the fires of inflammation, which is a common underpinning of many, if not all, chronic diseases and disorders. In fact, researchers discovered that people who work the night shift have higher rates of cancer, and that's likely due to a combination of more stress hormones and lower melatonin levels.[5]

To help your child sleep better, make sure they are getting the correct number of hours of sleep. Marc Weissbluth, MD, in *Healthy Sleep Habits, Happy Child*, recommends that a child who is one to three years old get a total of 12 to 14 hours of sleep per day, three to six year olds 10 to 12 hours per day, and seven to 12 year olds 10 to 11 hours per day.

But that's not all: *When* your child goes to sleep is important as well. If your child has a late bedtime, then the "second wind" kicks in and the adrenals produce stress hormones to deal with the stress of staying awake later. This leads to lower function for dealing with other types of stress, so anyone with a late bedtime can be irritable or out of it, but a late bedtime can also lead to more symptoms of allergies, asthma and rashes because there is less cortisol available to control inflammation.

When my older son was a baby, he had trouble getting to sleep and staying asleep. I consulted a sleep counselor in New York City – yes, there is such a thing – and she recommended that I put my son to bed very early, which is what Dr. Weissbluth recommends in his book, too. I was shocked to discover that doing so made it far easier for him to fall asleep because I was working with his body's natural rhythm. Not only that, but he slept longer, which I think is a great thing. Our children need all they sleep they can get to help them detoxify and repair their sensitive and damaged nervous systems.

Children need to be in bed much earlier because they need to sleep longer; the younger they are, the earlier they need to be in bed. When my boys were babies, they were in bed by (gasp!) 5:30pm or 6:00pm. Now, at ages seven and nine,

---

5. Hansen, J., Light at night, shiftwork, and breast cancer risk, *J Natl Cancer Inst.* 2001 Oct 17;93(20):1513-5.

they're in bed by 7:30pm or 8:00pm. As a health coach, I constantly see young babies and toddlers put to bed at 9:00pm or 10:00pm; I see this with my sons' friends, too. These bedtimes are far too late. I understand that many times the child is kept awake because the dad works late and wants to spend some time with the child, but I've got to tell you that in this case, you need to put your foot down and do what's best for your child.

I recommend that your child not be exposed to any light from a screen (TV, tablet, phone or computer) within one hour of bedtime because the blue light from screens can over-stimulate your child's pineal gland, which controls circadian rhythm and makes melatonin[6]. Blue-blocking lights – they're orange – are a great choice for the bedroom if your child needs a nightlight. Otherwise, keep the room as dark as possible, because exposure to light at night is linked to depression and learning disabilities because it halts the production and release of melatonin[7].

I also recommend exposing your child to either no artificial lights or only blue-blocking lights within an hour of bedtime; this will send signals to the body that it's time for sleep. A consistent eating and bedtime schedule also helps.

If your child needs help falling asleep, try giving them magnesium, GABA and/or melatonin, although some people choose not to give their child melatonin because it is a hormone. You can also try homeopathic insomnia tablets or valerian root tincture Speak with your practitioner about dosages that are right for your child.

If your child needs help staying asleep, try giving them glycine, an inhibitory neurotransmitter and amino acid that promotes delta-wave sleep.

If you're looking for a food-based approach to your child's sleep issues, here are my top 10 foods for a better night's sleep:

---

6. http://www.health.harvard.edu/newsletters/Harvard_Health_Letter/2012/May/blue-light-has-a-dark-side/. Accessed September 1, 2014.
7. Johns Hopkins. "Exposure to light at night may cause depression, learning issues, mouse study suggests." *ScienceDaily*. November 14, 2012.

- **Bone broth** is full of glycine and necessary minerals like magnesium. In fact, one tablespoon of powdered gelatin, which comes from bone broth, contains over 19,000mg of glycine!
- **Spinach** contains 690mg of tryptophan per cup.
- **Chia seeds** provide 721mg of tryptophan per cup of dried seeds.
- **Pig ears** have 4,400mg of glycine per ear. Don't cringe – they're a Vietnamese and Chinese delicacy!
- **Cherry tomatoes** are rich in GABA.
- **Kefir** contains GABA as well as probiotics if your child can tolerate fermented dairy.
- **Pumpkin seeds** provide 535mg of magnesium per cup.
- **Flax seeds** contain 392mg of magnesium per cup.
- **Mung beans** have 267mg of magnesium per cup of raw beans.
- **Buckwheat** provides 231mg of magnesium per cup, uncooked.

You'll also want to remove electronic devices from your child's room to improve sleep. A study by the National Sleep Foundation found that 75% of children have some form of electronic device in their room at night. If the devices are left on, children get, on average, an hour less of sleep.[8] There are a couple of possible reasons for this. One, lights and sounds from alerts could be continually waking the child. Two, if the device is not on airplane mode, studies have shown that the electromagnetic fields (EMF) of the device interferes with the ability to sleep.[9]

That's likely because chronic exposure to electromagnetic fields – whether from the device or Wi-Fi or a large electrical device such as a refrigerator – puts your child's body in a state of stress, even when resting. Research shows EMF can cause changes in both the sympathetic nervous system as well as the

---

8. www.sciencedaily.com/releases/2014/09/140904183554.htm. Accessed September 5, 2014.
9. http://www.ursi.org/proceedings/procGA08/papers/K02cp2.pdf. Accessed September 12, 2014.

parasympathetic nervous system by changing both the resting heart rate as well as heart-rate variability.[10]

Lowering Exposure to EMFs

It's almost impossible these days to completely eliminate your child's exposure to EMFs from cell phone, Wi-Fi, wireless devices and cell phone towers, but there are a lot of steps you can take to reduce exposure. Ann Louise Gittleman's book *Zapped: Why Your Cell Phone Shouldn't Be Your Alarm Clock and 1,268 Ways to Outsmart the Hazards of Electronic Pollution* shows you how to reduce your exposure while still being able to keep your electronics.

One tip is to make sure your child's bed isn't within a few feet, even on the other side of a wall, of a large electric device like a refrigerator or oven because these appliances generate large electromagnetic fields. You can also replace wireless phones with old-fashioned corded phones as well as replacing Wi-Fi with dial-up or at least turning your Wi Fi off at night. I always make sure to put my cell phone on airplane mode as much as possible, unless I'm using it and especially if the kids are playing on it or the iPad. Installing Stetzer filters and smart-meter cover are other great tips to lower the EMF burden on your child.

Grounding

The book *Earthing: The Most Important Health Discovery Ever?* by Clint Ober, Stephen T. Sinatra, MD and Martin Zucker makes a great case for how grounding can lower inflammation. Earthing is merely grounding, or ensuring that some uncovered part of your child's body is exposed to the

10. http://www.researchgate.net/publication/228993615_Provocation_study_using_heart_rate_variability_shows_microwave_radiation_from_2.4_GHz_cordless_phone_affects_autonomic_nervous_system. Accessed September 11, 2014.

earth to correct an electron deficiency, which can cause inflammation, sleep problems and stress.[11] It's the same principle that electricians use when they ground your house's electric system; they're simply attaching the entire system at some point to the ground on the outside of the house so that no excess charge builds up.

The easiest way to ground your child is to let him or her run around outside on an unpaved surface barefoot; just be sure it's in an area where pesticides haven't been applied. Wearing of rubber-soled shoes is one of the main ways that our children's bodies are cut off from the grounding energy of the earth.

Another way to ground your child – not in a punishment sense! – is to have your child sleep with a special grounding sheet or pillowcase that is attached to the ground of a nearby outlet. Also, make sure that when they're using an electronic device that they're touching a special grounding mat that is plugged into ground.

Yoga

Yoga is fairly well known for its ability to evoke a calming response in its practitioners. The smooth, slow integration of movement and breath calms the body as it quiets the mind. Long, deep breathing encourages the actions of the parasympathetic nervous system and allows more blood to flow to the digestive, reproductive, glandular, and immune systems.[12] Thus, healing is more likely to occur. These days, it's easy enough to find yoga classes for children; if you can't find one in your area, you can easily find DVDs that you can play at home.

---

11. Chevalier, G., Earthing: Health Implications of Reconnecting the Human Body to the Earth's Surface Electrons, *J Environ Public Health.* 2012; 2012: 291541.
12. Chandla, S.S., et al, Effect of short-term practice of pranayamic breathing exercises on cognition, anxiety, general well being and heart rate variability, *J Indian Med Assoc.* 2013 Oct;111(10):662-5.

Meditation and/or Prayer

Meditation and/or prayer can also calm your child because of the long, slow breathing involved. In addition, practicing these allows your child's mind to focus in a powerful way while learning how not to be distracted. If your child needs help in learning how to do this, there are plenty of podcasts and CDs of guided meditation that instruct your child how to relax the body while deepening the breath.

Pranayama Breathing

Dr. Andrew Weil taught me about pranayama breathing while I was attending the Institute for Integrative Nutrition. In a nutshell, it is a type of breath control taught in some yoga classes that stimulates the healing response of the parasympathetic nervous system. He calls one of these "relaxing breath (4-7-8),"[13] To do it, have your child breathe in through the nose for a count of four, hold for a count of seven, then exhale through the mouth while placing the tongue on the roof of the mouth for a count of eight. Do this for no more than four cycles.

Music

Playing soothing music can relax your SPD child. Much of Mozart's music is timed at 60 beats per minute, which would help to slow down the racing heart of an anxious or irritated child. One of the things I do when my sons get upset and have trouble calming down is to play Mozart, Bach or meditative music in their rooms. This is a pretty nice time out!

---

13. http://www.drweil.com/drw/u/ART00521/three-breathing-exercises.html. Accessed September 1, 2014.

Releasing Trapped Emotions

Trapped emotions can be a source of constant yet unacknowledged physical stress. Even infants can have trapped emotions because of a traumatic birth experience or emotions absorbed in utero. The Emotion Code and the Emotional Freedom Technique (EFT) are two types of painless therapies that your child can use to help break some of the emotional sources of anxiety.

Acupuncture

If your child is up for it, acupuncture is a very calming and ancient form of healing that is well-documented in its ability to reduce anxiety.[14] It seems like it wouldn't be because of having so many small needles inserted into the skin, but the truth is I always fall asleep during my acupuncture treatments.

Getting Outside

Children these days have what Richard Louv calls "nature deficit disorder." The lure of electronic devices is simply too great, yet it disconnects them from the free, healing benefits that come from being in nature. Being outside, whether it's playing on the beach, hiking a trail, playing on a swingset or playing ball, gives your child the ability to connect with natural cycles and rhythms, which is calming.

Skin Brushing

Typically, when your child starts seeing an occupational therapist for sensory integration, the OT will teach you how to

---

14. Mao, J.J., et al, Electroacupuncture for fatigue, sleep, and psychological distress in breast cancer patients with aromatase inhibitor-related arthralgia: A randomized trial, *Cancer.* 2014 Jul 30. doi: 10.1002/cncr.28917.

brush your child's skin with a surgical brush. It seems strange, but skin brushing helps your child calm down and organize his or her senses.

Joint Compression

Your OT will also likely show you how to do joint compression for your SPD child. Not only does this help your child know where his or her body is in space, but it is also a calming and organizing daily therapy for your child.

Amino Acid Therapy

Tryptophan is an amino acid that can be used to combat feelings of anxiety and depression, and it is far safer than an SSRI (selective serotonin reuptake inhibitor) anti-depressant. In fact, the U.S. Food and Drug Administration (FDA) has a "black box" label warning for the use of SSRI's because it can increase the risk of suicidal thinking and behavior in some children and adolescents. Anecdotally, all teenage perpetrators of mass shootings that I've heard about have been on some form of anti-depressant.

Other risks of SSRI's are:

- Insomnia
- Skin rashes
- Headaches
- Joint and muscle pain
- Stomach upset
- Nausea
- Diarrhea
- Stomach bleeding, especially if taking NSAIDs (aspirin, ibuprofen, naproxen)
- Tics
- Muscle spasms
- Repetitive muscle movements
- Compulsive restlessness

- Anxiety, which is ironic given that antidepressants are often given to people with anxiety

GABA is another amino acid that can help with feelings of anxiety; it's also a neurotransmitter.[15] It is an inhibitory neurotransmitter that counterbalances the action of the excitatory neurotransmitter glutamate.

It is important to note that another cause of amino-acid deficiency is low stomach acid. If your child doesn't have enough stomach acid, then he or she is not able to tear protein completely apart into its constituent amino acids. In addition, a child with gut dysbiosis may not be able to efficiently convert serotonin in the gut, where most of it is made.

Essential Oils

Several essential oils can have a calming effect and lower the response of the sympathetic nervous system;[16] the most commonly known are lavender,[17] chamomile and valerian, although there are several others such as orange, tangerine, jasmine, bergamot, rose, clary sage, lemon, pine, geranium, marjoram and sandalwood. In addition, there are quite a few blends sold by various companies that are specifically designed to reduce anxiety.

Five Smells a Day

The Family Hope Center in Norristown, PA recommends having your child smell five different scents a day as a way of opening up parts of the brain that are neurodevelopmentally

---

15. Lydiard RB, The role of GABA in anxiety disorders, *J Clin Psychiatry*. 2003;64 Suppl 3:21-7.
16. Haze, S., et al, Effects of fragrance inhalation on sympathetic activity in normal adults, *Jpn J Pharmacol*. 2002 Nov;90(3):247-53.
17. Lee, I.S., Effects of lavender aromatherapy on insomnia and depression in women college students, *Taehan Kanho Hakhoe Chi*. 2006 Feb;36(1):136-43.

damaged.[18] Smells activate the amygdala, which controls memory, decision-making and emotional reactions and hippocampus, which processes emotion, and bypass the higher cortical areas, which process reasoning and logic.

Healing the Adrenals and Thyroid

The key to lowering the stress response for your SPD child is healing the adrenals and thyroid, which are linked in controlling the body's response to stress. Typically, if a person has adrenal problems, they also have thyroid problems; there is roughly an 80% overlap.

Stress chews up valuable minerals that are needed for proper adrenal and thyroid function. Therefore, getting minerals into your child is essential to lowering his or her stress response, but I recommend starting with food-based sources of minerals first: bone broth, unrefined salt, vegetables, seaweed and liver or other animal organs before supplementing. The use of adaptogenic herbs can also be a gentle way to modulate feelings of anxiety, and, in my opinion, should be used before working with your child's doctor for adrenal and/or thyroid extract supplementation.

Lowering your child's stress response lowers inflammation and the need for cortisol in your child's body. Doing this will thus help with sensory processing problems from neuroinflammation as well as mood swings, tantrums and some behavioral issues because cortisol also controls blood sugar.

Bone Broth

Bone broth is one of the staples in my kitchen, and I'm hoping to make it that way in yours, too. Our ancestors knew about bone broth benefits, but we've gotten so out of touch

18. http://vimeo.com/93286354. Accessed September 2, 2014.

with traditional foods that we don't realize how healing something as simple as bone broth can be.

"Good broth will resurrect the dead" is a South American proverb. The reason is that animal bones are full of minerals. So many people are mineral deficient these days, especially those who eat a Standard American Diet full of processed foods that are typically void of vitamins, minerals and other nutrients. Minerals are necessary for proper functioning of our adrenal and thyroid glands, which help us to deal with stress. If your child is mineral deficient, and most SPD kids are, he or she is likely having a hard time managing stress.

When broth cools, the gelatin in it congeals. Gelatin contains the amino acids glycine and arginine. Glycine is helpful for achieving deep, restful sleep as well as for making glutathione, the body's master antioxidant. Arginine helps heal coronary blood vessels, keeps the plaque off of arteries and minimizes clotting.

Gelatin also helps heal the lining of the colon, and is especially helpful for digestive issues that your child likely has. In addition, gelatin is anti-inflammatory, so it can help reduce the anxiety stress response that your SPD child has.

Bone broth is the magic ingredient I use to give my home-cooked meals a satisfying and rich flavor. Anyone that's eaten my food knows that it has a deep, hearty richness that comes from my homemade bone broths. You can't buy this flavor from a package in a store or even find it in most restaurants, as they use factory-made bases containing MSG or other free-glutamate "foods". You really need to make it yourself to taste the difference. You can use bone broth for reconstituting grains and legumes, for sautéing and braising meats and vegetables and for the base for sauces and soups.

Be sure to use bones from pasture-raised or grass-fed land animals or from wild-caught (not farm-raised) fish. When you buy meat, be sure to buy it with the bone in and skin on. Fat from the skin is full of fat-soluble vitamins and gives dishes another depth of flavor that's impossible to duplicate with store- or restaurant-bought food. Save the bones and store them in the freezer until you have enough to make a batch of bone broth in your slow cooker.

Unrefined Salt

Unrefined salt is an excellent source of minerals, especially trace minerals. Your child's craving for sweet or salty foods can be a sign that his or her adrenals need support in the form of minerals. Despite what we've been led to believe, salt IS good for your health but not the sodium-laden, refined table salt that people commonly use these days.

Don't believe me? The Weston A. Price Foundation's article "The Salt of the Earth" is a great source of information about the health benefits of salt and the important role it plays in our metabolism, digestion, brain function and adrenal health.[19] Another great resource is David Brownstein's book, *Salt: Why You Need It, Why You Can't Live Without It.* In addition, recent research has found no link between salt consumption and an increased risk of death or cardiovascular disease,[20] so let's lay that fear to rest.

When I say "salt," I mean it has to be an unrefined, naturally colored land or sea salt, not white, refined common salt. Himalayan salt, Celtic sea salt and Redmond's Real Salt are all good examples of unrefined salt. Use as much unrefined salt as tastes good to your child. You can even put it in a little water for a pick-me-up.

Vegetables

Vegetables are an excellent source of minerals. Annemarie Colbin, founder of the Natural Gourmet Institute in New York City, says when someone asks her about where to

---

19. http://www.westonaprice.org/health-topics/abcs-of-nutrition/the-salt-of-the-earth/. Accessed August 31, 2014.
20. McCarron, David A., Dietary sodium and cardiovascular and renal disease risk factors: dark horse or phantom entry?, *Nephrol Dial Transplant.* Jul 2008; 23(7): 2133–2137.

get calcium if you're dairy-free, "Where do you think the cows get it from? Or horses? Or sheep? They get it from eating grass and plants." Your child can, too, so be sure to offer lots of vegetables to your child. You can also make a vegetable broth or add vegetables to your bone broth, then use the broth for drinking by itself or cooking soups, grains and legumes.

Seaweed

Seaweed is an unsung hero, yet it's so full of essential minerals, especially iodine, which is necessary for the health of the thyroid and reproductive organs and glands. If your child says, "Oooh, yuck!" at the thought of eating seaweed – and I don't mean the neon green seaweed salads sold in Asian restaurants – add in strips of kombu (kelp) to soups, grains and legumes that you're cooking. You can remove the kombu after cooking if you like; its minerals will have leached out into the rest of the food.

Liver and Other Organs

Animal organs are extremely high in minerals; just make sure you buy pasture-raised or, at the very least, organic versions, so it's a good idea to eat animal organs like liver at least once a week like your grandparents used to. This is one of the hardest things to get my clients to do! I find that cooking liver with a lot of onions helps to mask the gamey flavor of it.

Cooking Fruits and Vegetables

Health coach and *Top Chef* contender Andrea Beaman recommends that people with adrenal fatigue not eat raw food, as this requires more energy from the body than people with adrenal fatigue have. This means even cooking your fruit. Try sautéing your fruit in ghee or coconut oil and cinnamon with the lid on over low heat; it's delicious!

Magnesium Supplementation

The Magnesium Miracle by Carolyn Dean, MD, ND, is an easy-to-read, yet informative book about the many ways that magnesium helps our body's processes, yet is so often missing from our diets. Most people are deficient in this critical nutrient, and our SPD kids are in huge need of it to help calm them down. Magnesium supplementation can be a great way to deal with stress; stress and sugar consumption use up magnesium tremendously. Remember that sugar IS stress to your child's body, as it causes inflammation.

Magnesium calms the central nervous system, and it also helps lower your child's incidences of asthma and allergies. Supplementation with it can help your child go to sleep as well as help with middle-of-the-night insomnia. Magnesium can also help with constipation and/or chronic diarrhea, which is typically the flip side of chronic constipation, as it is taken to "bowel tolerance," meaning if you get to the point where your child's stools are too loose, like diarrhea, then back off the dosage a bit.

The best forms are magnesium citramate, magnesium citrate and magnesium glycinate. Magnesium oxide is the form most commonly found in supermarket and drugstore brands, but it's very ineffective in my experience. Magnesium chelate is another common form, but "chelate" is a meaningless term because it just means "chemically bound to something else," and, in this case, we don't know what that something else is.

Zinc Supplementation

A small amount of zinc is necessary for proper function of both the thyroid and immune system, and it is also an antioxidant, meaning it can calm inflammation as well as anxiety. A deficiency of zinc is linked to fatigue and an inability to focus. Supplementing with small doses of zinc can expand your child's sense of taste and smell, helping them to overcome their picky eating habits. I prefer zinc in the form of zinc glycinate.

Iodine Supplementation

Iodine is necessary for proper thyroid function, and it has a profound effect on the body's immune system. The best way to get more iodine into your child is by putting kelp/kombu into soups, stews, beans, lentils when cooking. I don't recommend iodized salt because the versions that I've seen are typically refined salt that has been iodized.

Selenium Supplementation

Selenium is another mineral that's essential in small doses for the health of your child's thyroid. Brazil nuts are famous for their selenium content, but don't let your child eat them like crazy. Work with your practitioner to get the proper dosage. Just be sure that neither selenium selenite nor selenium selenate are given because these are toxic byproducts, yet they are the forms commonly found in most grocery-store and pharmacy brands.[21]

Methyl Supplementation

Your child can get methyl groups straight from the source: leafy greens. The words folic and folate come from "foliage", as in leaves. Green juices and green-juice powders are excellent sources of natural folate. Methylated forms of folate in supplement form are:

---

21. http://www.greenmedinfo.com/blog/your-multivitamin-toxic-0. Accessed September 1, 2014.

- L (L-5-methyltetrahydrofolate (L-5-MTHF))
- 6S,
- Quatrofolic or
- Metafolin; L-5-methyltetrahydrofolate (L-5-MTHF)

I don't recommend taking supplements willy nilly because if your child takes the wrong form or the wrong amount, he or she may experience side effects. For targeted supplement advice, you can have your child work with:

- A naturopath
- A functional-medicine doctor
- Dr. Ben Lynch of MTHFR.net, or
- Dr. Amy Yasko. Dr. Yasko has developed the "Yasko Protocol" which is a targeted supplement protocol that varies depending on which genetic mutations your child has. You can find out more about it on her website: www.dramyyasko.com.

Vitamin D Supplementation

Sherry Rogers, MD, says that optimal levels are over 80, despite the fact that 30 to 70 is considered "normal." If levels are low, you'll need to supplement – just be sure it's vitamin D_3, not D_2 which is synthetic and is often found in foods saying "contains vitamin D". Also, having your child supplement with vitamin K_2 as well as eat plenty of fat helps activate these fat-soluble vitamins. *NOTE: All forms of vitamin K may interact with blood thinning medications. If your child is taking such medicines, please consult with your physician before having your child take this product.*

Adaptogenic Herbs

Adaptogenic herbs can calm the central nervous and adrenal systems. Holy basil and ashwaganda (in small doses) can be used for calming anxiety. For further information about this subject, you can read, *Adaptogens: Herbs for Strength, Stamina and Stress Relief*, by David Winston and Steven Maimes. Consider supplementing with adaptogenic herbs if the lifestyle changes, food and supplements I discussed aren't sufficient in boosting your child's energy and lowering irritability and sensory issues. You may want to have an Adrenal Stress Profile test performed by your functional-medicine or naturopathic doctor first.

Adrenal Extracts

If you find that lifestyle changes, food, supplements and adaptogenic herbs still aren't making enough of a difference, ask your practitioner to run an Adrenal Cortex Stress Profile test. If your child's cortisol levels are low, your practitioner may be able to offer your child adrenal extracts, which are bioidentical, dried adrenal glands of cows, pigs and sheep.

Thyroid Extracts

Your child may also need thyroid extracts, if testing and body temperature warrant. Thyroid extracts are also bioidentical hormones that come from thyroid glands of cows or pigs; it's usually called "Armour" and can be a little tricky to dose. For more information on this subject, read *Stop the Thyroid Madness* by Janie A. Bowthorpe.

Other Thyroid Issues

There are quite a few lifestyle changes that you can make to lower the effect of endocrine disruptors on your child's thyroid:

- Switch to a fluoride-free toothpaste.
- Avoid anything that says "anti-bacterial" if it has triclosan in it. Triclosan is a pesticide that damages the thyroid as well.

- Get rid of as much plastic in your life and replace with glass or stainless steel. This includes water and juices bought in plastic bottles.
- Get rid of your Teflon® and non-stick cookware and replace with cast iron, glass and/or enamel cookware.
- Avoid unfermented soy and *raw* goitrogenic foods such as broccoli, cauliflower, cabbage, bok choy, kale and spinach. This means NO juiced kale or spinach, too!
- Avoid gluten, which is found in wheat, barley, rye and oats that are not certified as being gluten free. Millet, even though it is gluten-free, can have a thyroid-suppressive effect, too.

Lowering Inflammation

Having your child eat anti-inflammatory, antioxidant foods is a great way to control inflammation and thus lower anxiety and sensory problems. Loading up with minerals through eating animal organs like liver, eating vegetables, sea vegetables and broth and supplementing with minerals, especially magnesium, will help support the adrenals and thus control inflammation.

Eating no-added-sugar foods and eliminating processed foods helps your child's body manage blood-sugar swings that can lead to inflammation. Remember that sugar is the most inflammatory food around; I would say that vegetable oils, which are rancid from processing, are the second most.

Increase Antioxidants

"Eating the rainbow" provides your child with high levels of naturally occurring antioxidants and other phytonutrients. Following is a non-exhaustive list of naturally colorful foods:

- **Red foods:** radishes, beets, strawberries, tomatoes, red bell peppers, goji berries, red onions
- **Orange foods:** oranges, kumquats, persimmons, apricots,

orange bell peppers, sweet potatoes, carrots
- **Yellow foods:** summer squash, bananas, yellow apples
- **Green foods:** kale, cucumbers, zucchini, cabbage, celery, cilantro, parsley, mustard greens, lettuce, turnip greens, artichokes, asparagus, scallions
- **Blue foods:** blueberries
- **Purple foods:** red cabbage, eggplants
- **Black foods:** wild rice
- **White foods:** cauliflower, potatoes, Hannah yams, onions, garlic

Cooking with fresh herbs such as rosemary, oregano, cilantro and parsley as well as spices such as turmeric, garlic and ginger can lower your child's inflammation because these foods are also loaded with antioxidants.

Consult with your practitioner about having your child supplement with various antioxidants such as vitamin C, vitamin A and vitamin E. Vitamin C is especially helpful, as this water-soluble vitamin helps your child's body recycle glutathione, the body's master antioxidant.

Eliminate Processed Foods

Stress and food choice can be like a chicken-or-the-egg game: which came first? Processed food can exacerbate stress, and stress can lead to processed food cravings. When I say "processed food," I mean anything that comes in a bag, box or can. I also mean 99% of all restaurant food and prepared foods because these typically contain ingredients that I don't consider healthy, such as added sugars, preservatives, additives, canola oil, soy oil or other vegetable oils.

Processed foods typically contain refined sugars/carbohydrates and refined oils, two of the most unhealthy "foods" there are. Not only do they cause inflammation, which is a key component of any chronic health condition like Sensory Processing Disorder, but they also cause reactive hypoglycemia, which stresses your child's adrenal glands, which reduces their ability to handle stress and lower inflammation, which means they crave carby/bready/sugary foods that can raise your blood sugar quickly. It's a vicious cycle.

In addition to being nutritionally deficient, these "foods" also cause nutritional deficiencies in order to metabolize them. It takes something like 50 molecules of magnesium to process one molecule of sugar. With Americans consuming 130 POUNDS of sugar every year, it's no wonder most people are magnesium deficient these days! Magnesium is a critical mineral that is essential for relaxing the central nervous system.

So here's what you do: once or twice a week, cook a big batch of something that's easy to throw together, like chili or stew. Eat half during the week, and freeze the other half for later. Do the same with whole grains, like brown rice or quinoa; you can freeze whole grains, too.

Every day, you'll need to cook fresh vegetables. Sounds hard, but it's not, and it really doesn't take too much time. My favorite ways for cooking them quickly are roasting with a little olive oil and sea salt, steaming or sautéing with garlic, olive oil and sea salt. You can find a few more recipes in the back of this book.

Try this for a week or two, and see if your child doesn't feel better. Eating whole foods can help your child handle stress a whole lot better.

Cut Out Sugar

A key part of recovering your child from Sensory Processing Disorder is to cut our sugar in all of its forms such as cane sugar, high fructose corn syrup, maple syrup and rice syrup. Even fruit juice on its own counts as sugar because that's really all it is. The reason to cut out sugar is that blood-sugar swings caused by too much sugar wear out your child's adrenals and leave him or her less able to deal effectively with processing sensory stimuli.

However, telling you to cut out sugar in your child's diet is much easier than you doing it because sugar is as addictive as drugs! Sugar activates the same pleasure centers in the brain that hard drugs like morphine and heroin do, and your child get a dopamine rush from consuming it. No wonder it's so hard to give up.

Giving up sugar is hard, and sheer willpower probably won't be enough to do it. I've found that cutting out processed foods while adding in more fat and foods made from scratch and whole grains helps. Let me be clear on what I mean by "made from whole grains." I mean food made with the whole brown rice, millet, quinoa, oats grain/kernel, not flakes or flour made by grinding up these grains and seeds. I mean food made with the whole wheat berry, if you eat wheat, not bread or cookies or waffles or pancakes made from whole wheat flour. I mean whole oat groats, not oatmeal. Grinding a grain into flour increases its glycemic load, meaning it can raise your child's blood sugar very quickly.

Soda, in my opinion, is one of THE most dangerous foods around these days. Please don't let your child drink it. Not only does soda contain no nutrients, it's loaded with ingredients that are making your child's sensory symptoms worse. I recommend that your child drink water instead.

Get Rid of Vegetable Oils and Trans Fats

Hopefully, you don't have any Crisco or margarine, even if it's soy margarine or some other allegedly "heart healthy" solidified vegetable oil spreads. If you do have them, throw them out! They are full of trans fats, which are indeed the most dangerous of all fats. Even tiny amounts raise the risk of heart disease. This also means to eliminate processed foods because they typically contain hydrogenated vegetable oils to keep them shelf-stable for long periods of time. Good food SHOULD be able to rot!

In addition, throw out any vegetable oils such as soy oil, corn oil, canola oil or Wesson from your cabinets because these vegetable oils are highly inflammatory, and some, such as canola oil, are mostly trans fat due to the amount of processing they undergo.

Cook with Saturated Fats or EVOO

Many of the foods that we were led to believe are "healthy" are not. We've been duped by Big Ag's marketing campaigns for decades. Saturated fats have been demonized, while vegetable oils have been praised. This couldn't be further from the truth, as the British Medical Journal,[22] the Weston A. Price Foundation[23] and Udo Erasmus in *Fats That Heal, Fats That Kill* explain.

Saturated fats should be used for cooking because their high-strength (saturated) bonds don't break under typical cooking temperatures and, therefore, do not become rancid and inflammatory. For cooking, use extra-virgin olive oil (EVOO) or saturated fats that your grandmother used to use, such as:

- Ghee
- Butter (if your child can tolerate dairy)
- Coconut oil (whose medium chain fatty acids are particularly helpful for neurological disorders)
- Schmaltz (chicken fat)
- Lard (pork fat)
- Tallow (beef fat)
- Duck fat

Supplement with Essential Fatty Acids

SPD kids are notoriously deficient in essential fatty acids (EFAs), especially omega-3 fatty acids. EFAs calm inflammation and the central nervous system, and numerous studies have shown that they help reduce symptoms of

---

22. Malhotra, A., Saturated fat is not the major issue, *BMJ* 2013;347:f6340
23. http://www.westonaprice.org/health-topics/the-oiling-of-america/. Accessed September 1, 2014.

ADHD, autism, allergies, and asthma, as these are all chronic diseases with chronic inflammation in common.

Armed with the results of the NutrEval, CardioIon, BodyBio or other targeted tests your practitioner offers, you'll be able to know which fatty acids your child is deficient in. SPD kids are typically deficient in DHA, which is necessary for brain health and can be found in cod liver oil; cod liver oil also contains EPA, which helps more with general inflammation.

My friend, Dan Corrigan, the founder of Corganic, a company that sells specialized nutritional supplements for neurodevelopmentally damaged kids, says to be careful of the quality of cod liver oil. Because of the way it's processed, it can go rancid (become inflammatory) very quickly. The Weston A. Price Foundation recommends fermented cod liver oil, but, after traveling to Norway and working with cod fishermen, Dan learned that fermented cod liver oil goes rancid quickly, as well.

In addition to supplementing with cod liver oil, you'll want to target other fatty acid deficiencies. Even if your child isn't deficient in other fatty acids, it's a good idea to rotate other beneficial fatty acids like evening primrose oil, hemp oil, flax oil and walnut oil. Many SPD kids lack the ability to convert these other fatty acids into DHA and EPA, so be sure your child takes them in addition to cod liver oil. Just be sure to refrigerate all of these, as they are very fragile and can go rancid quickly.

Do an Elimination Diet

Allergenic foods cause inflammation, and when the body has inflammation, it starts attacking itself and anything it perceives as attacking it, like pollen or cat dander. This is known as an autoimmune attack and can lead to any number of illnesses, but for children, they usually show up as eczema, allergies, asthma, ADHD and/or autism.

Having your child eliminate the following top allergenic foods for one week, then add them back in one at a time is the gold standard for identifying hidden sources of inflammation:

- Gluten (wheat, barley, rye and non-gluten free oats)
- Dairy (such as milk, cheese, cream cheese, sour cream)
- Corn (be sure to avoid non-pasture-raised beef, pork and eggs, as they are generally fed corn and soy)
- Soy (tofu, tempeh, miso, soy sauce, etc. Be VERY careful with processed foods as many seemingly "healthy" foods contain soy in many of its varied forms. Read the list of ingredients for hidden soy like soy protein isolate, textured vegetable protein and natural and artificial flavorings.)
- Eggs
- Nuts
- Shellfish
- Fish

During the elimination week, your child can eat the following instead of gluten-containing foods:

- Rice
- Potatoes
- Millet
- Buckwheat
- Quinoa
- Sweet potatoes
- Chickpeas
- Amaranth
- Sorghum
- Teff
- Lentils
- Any type of bean

Then reintroduce the potential allergens one by one every 4 days. Be sure to keep a food journal for any adverse or unusual reactions upon reintroduction such as:

- Headaches
- Stomach pain
- Foggy thinking

- Irritability
- Rashes

If you find that your child is sensitive to gluten and/or dairy, which is typical for SPD kids, as well as for children with autism and ADHD, I'll be discussing the elimination of those foods later in the book.

Cross-Reactivity

If your child shows sensitivity to certain allergenic foods, you need to be aware that some foods can cause cross-reactions. For example, gluten can cross react with corn, dairy and oats, meaning that if your child is sensitive to gluten, it's a good idea to remove these foods as well. Or, children with a soy allergy may need to avoid peanuts and other legumes.

Do a Rotation Diet

Consider a rotation diet, which can be used to keep from developing sensitivities to foods. For example, if your child had an IgG test done or did an elimination diet, and it shows that they should avoid gluten and eggs, you'll of course have your child avoid gluten and eggs.

What typically happens, though, is that parents get into a rut with their child's diets and offer the same things day in and day out. So even though your child is avoiding gluten and eggs, they can build up sensitivities to the other foods that they're eating consistently to avoid gluten and eggs, especially if they have leaky gut, which these kids typically do. What you need is a rotation diet that doesn't give your child's body enough time to build up sensitivities to newly introduced foods.

My best advice is to keep it simple and don't make any complicated recipes. That way it's easier to keep track of which ingredients are legal for the particular days of the diet your child is on. Roasting and steaming are two very easy ways to prepare foods, especially vegetables, without making it complicated.

Check for Other Food Sensitivities

If your child's issues could use more improvement, but you've hit a plateau with the dietary changes you've made so far, it's time to check into further food sensitivities. Oxalates, glutamates, histamines, salicylates, phenols, nightshades and FODMAP foods are groups of foods that could be causing hidden food sensitivities.

Oxalates

Foods with high levels of oxalates can contribute to inflammation if your child still has a leaky gut, deepening the level of gut dysbiosis. Many foods contain some level of oxalates, so the key here is to avoid ones with high levels, such as spinach, Swiss chard, parsley, almonds, cashews, most beans, wheat, buckwheat, many types of berries, celery, sweet potatoes and chocolate. Julie Matthews' book, *Nourishing Hope for Autism: Nutrition and Diet Guide for Healing Children: ADHD, Autism, Learning and Developmental Delays*, is an excellent resource for learning more about avoiding these foods.

Glutamates

Monsodium glutamate is the most well-known free glutamate, and it's an excitoxin, which means it stimulates brain cells to the point of cell death. Translation: eat MSG and kill your brain. Free glutamates, which are found in most processed foods as well as some non-processed foods such as whey protein and soy protein, can cause sensory and behavioral problems in children and is linked to neurological disorders like Parkinson's, Alzheimer's, ALS and more. I don't see the ALS Association talking about that on their website or in their ice-bucket challenges.

I highly recommend that you check out the work of Dr. Katherine Reid, founder of Unblind My Mind and biochemist, who recovered her daughter from autism simply by removing free glutamates from her food. I have a client whose son shed many of his autistic symptoms as well when free glutamates were removed from his diet.

I've noticed that very few products these days actually use outright MSG, although I was shocked when I read the ingredients list on a bag of Dorito's and found it listed MSG right there for everyone to see. Instead, what you typically see is "soy protein isolate," "autolyzed yeast extract," "textured vegetable protein" or other concoctions. In addition, foods like corn starch, corn syrup, vinegars and other commonly found ingredients can trigger MSG reactions in sensitive people.[24]

Histamines

One of the roles of histamines is to create inflammatory attacks, which cause blood vessels to swell. If your child's body doesn't process histamines well, he or she might build up an intolerance to them. Symptoms such as headache, anxiety, abdominal pain, nausea, nasal congestion, hives and flushing can all be signs of a histamine intolerance. Examples of high-histamine foods are avocado, aged cheese, citrus fruit, chocolate, pork, fermented foods like vinegar and sauerkraut, spinach, strawberries and processed meats. Try eliminating these foods for a week to see if your child's symptoms improve.

Phenols and Salicylates

Children with low levels of the enzyme phenol-sulfotransferase-P can't process phenols and salicylates well;

---

24. http://www.truthinlabeling.org/hiddensources.html. Accessed September 5, 2014.

many children with autism, ADHD and Sensory Processing Disorder have insufficient levels of this enzyme. Sensitivity to foods containing high levels of phenols and salicylates can cause your child to have dark circles under the eyes, hyperactivity, red cheeks or ears after eating, aggressiveness, difficulty sleeping and inappropriate laughter.

The Feingold diet was developed by Ben Feingold to remove high levels of these foods from the diet, as well as artificial colors, artificial flavors, artificial sweeteners and preservatives. Most foods have some level of them, so the trick is to remove the ones with high levels such as berries, apples, oranges, grapes and raisins. For more information about this, check out the Feingold Association of the United States' website at www.feingold.org

Nightshades

Although nightshades are common foods in the Western diet, they can cause pain and inflammation in a person with an intolerance for them. These foods are tomatoes, potatoes, bell peppers, spicy peppers, paprika and eggplant. Tobacco is another nightshade plant. It takes about six weeks for nightshades to completely leave the body, so you'll need to eliminate them from your child's diet for that long before reintroducing for a challenge. Sherry Rogers, MD's book *Pain Free in Six Weeks* is a great resource about this subject.

FODMAP

FODMAP is an acronym for Fermentable Oligosaccharides, Disaccharides, Monosaccharides And Polyols. These are short-chain carbohydrates that aren't completely absorbed in the gut; thus, they tend to ferment and cause intestinal distress. Many common foods are high-FODMAP foods. Examples of them are garlic, onions, apples, wheat, pistachios, honey and most dairy products. The website www.fodmaps.com is a great resource for those wanting to learn more.

Try BioSET, NAET or the Ellen Cutler Method

There is an easier way to deal with food and other sensitivities, if you have the access, and that is to visit a BioSET, NAET (Namudripad's Allergy Elimination Techniques) or Ellen Cutler Method practitioner (see Resources for websites). They are similar holistic approaches that incorporate acupressure, energy healing, immunology, enzyme therapy and nutrition to assist the body's natural healing process in eliminating sensitivities. Because these techniques use muscle testing or electro-dermal screening for identifying sensitivities, it may be a little too out there for most parents. I encourage you to keep an open mind, try it, and see if the system helps your child or not before judging it. I know far too many people that this type of identification works for, including myself.

Allergies, not just outright, anaphylactic allergies and runny noses, but sensitivities to just about anything can lead to a multitude of seemingly unrelated symptoms like headaches, depression, fatigue, hyperactivity, digestive problems and asthma. Many people may not understand that their children have sensitivities to foods and chemicals in their environment. SPD kids can develop sensitivities to their own hormones and even nutrients like vitamins, minerals and essential fatty acids. Dr. Ellen Cutler tells us that having a sensitivity to hormones or nutrients causes a deficiency of them.[25] Interesting!

The use of digestive enzymes to improve digestive function, which is the basis of health, and the use of these allergy-elimination techniques to clear children from sensitivities can relieve them from symptoms of Sensory

---

25. Cutler, Ellen, DC, *Clearing the Way to Health and Wellness: Reversing Chronic Conditions by Freeing the Body of Food, Environmental, and Other Sensitivities.* Bloomington, IN: iUniverse, 2013, 83.

Processing Disorder, as well as various health conditions such as sinus infections, hay fever, Chronic Fatigue Immune Disorder Syndrome (CFIDS), fibromyalgia, *Candida* yeast infections, Chron's disease, ulcerative colitis, hypothyroidism and Hashimoto's thyroiditis.

Controlling Blood Sugar Swings

Blood-sugar swings wear out your child's adrenals. Sugar is inflammatory, and cortisol made by the adrenal glands is needed to lower the inflammation, thereby leaving less cortisol available for dealing with stress and chronic inflammation. Cortisol also controls your child's circadian rhythm. The result of having low cortisol can be a child that is cranky, irritable, gets sick a lot, has trouble sleeping and has trouble understanding what their senses are telling them.

Adding more fat to your child's diet can help control blood sugar and thus reduce the need for cortisol. Adding more avocado to your child's diet is a great way to start, such as with the Creamy Fruit Pudding Without the Cream recipe in the back of the book. Grains, sugars and starches, especially processed ones – and this means anything made with "flour" except for coconut, nut or seed flours – have higher glycemic indexes and thus elevate blood sugar. Focus on adding more fiber from legumes, vegetables and fruit, as well as protein and fat. Just be sure to cook the fruits and vegetables first.

Having your child eat foods that are high in protein, fat and fiber can help tremendously as well as having them avoid foods that are high in sugar and processed carbs will help manage their blood sugar. You may think most store-bought yogurt is good for your kids, but have you ever looked at the nutritional label? Most of them are loaded with sugar, and that sugar will contribute to hypoglycemia, an insatiable need for processed carbs and sugar, sensory sensitivities, and an inability to control angry outbursts.

Eating carbohydrates by themselves contributes to hypoglycemic issues, so make sure your child has a source of unprocessed protein with every meal and with many of their snacks. Beef jerky, hummus, bean dips and nuts are great protein-rich snacks.

Test Blood Sugar

If your child can tolerate being tested, I recommend getting a home blood testing kit so you can check your child's fasting and non-fasting blood sugar levels. You can find testing kits on Amazon for as low as $15. It's not the meter that's expensive, though; it's the strips. Your child may show a blood-sugar sensitivity to certain foods or combinations of foods.

If you find that your child's non-fasting blood sugar is over 140 a half hour after eating, first try working in more fat to the meal or snack with the suspected offending food next time; fasting levels before breakfast should be no higher than 100, although 85 is a better result. If your child continues to show blood-sugar sensitivity, remove that food from the diet for a few weeks, then reintroduce with a challenge, keeping note of blood-sugar spikes as well as physical and behavioral problems. Allergy-elimination techniques such as BioSET, NAET and the Ellen Cutler Method can remove the sensitivity.

Using Therapies for Sensory Integration

Typically, your child will begin working with an occupational therapist (OT) for correcting sensory issues. However, there are a few things to keep in mind:

- Having your child receive cranioscacral therapy first can lessen the time involved with other therapies.
- Having your child receive vision therapy before other therapies except for craniosacral therapy can lead to huge gains and can lessen the time with other therapies.
- Simultaneously implementing the advice I just discussed about lowering stress, healing the adrenals and thyroid and

lowering inflammation will improve your child's outcome with any therapy.
- Many OTs don't understand how to integrate primitive reflexes. Addressing these needs with therapies like Rhythmic Movement Training, the Masgutova Method or other primitive-reflex integration therapy before moving onto traditional sensory diets can improve your child's outcome faster.

Try Craniosacral Therapy

Patricia Lemer recommends craniosacral therapy (CST) as the number two thing you should do for SPD kids. (Number one is reducing the stress of a toxic load, which is what I've been teaching you how to do.)

Craniosacral therapy is an extremely gentle therapy that's typically performed by a chiropractor. It's very relaxing. It may not look like the practitioner is doing much except for giving your child a head message, but there's a good chance your child will be more calm and less stressed after having a CST session. Remember: the key to recovery is lowering stress.

Get a Vision Therapy Assessment

It's essential that you get your child's eyes checked by a developmental optometrist (you can find one at www.covd.org). Patricia Lemer is adamant about this, and I am, too, after discovering that many autistic behaviors such as stimming, flapping arms, lining up cars, sideways glancing, and social unresponsiveness are CAUSED by vision problems. Vision is not the same thing as seeing, so don't expect that a typical optometrist or ophthalmologist will know about this.

Think about it: vision uses up about 80% of the bandwidth of the nervous system, so reducing visual stress reduces the overall stress load on the body. Many children become more verbal or social pretty quickly after beginning vision therapy, while allergies, sickness and sleeping improve.

Just be sure that the optometrist runs an Irlen diagnostic test, which means that the optometrist places a long series of colored lenses over your child's eyes, then asks him or her to look at different things in the room. Children with vision problems will often see letters and words dance or fall off the page. Imagine the strain and fatigue of your child trying to read if this is happening! After performing an Irlen test, the optometrist may prescribe tinted lenses that help correct this kind of visual processing problem.

I am fortunate to have Dr. Randy Schulman, MS, OD, FCOVD, as my sons' behavioral optometrist. Dr. Schulman wrote the chapters on the role of vision therapy and optometry in Patricia Lemer's first book, *Envisioning a Bright Future: Interventions that Work for Children and Adults with Autism Spectrum Disorders*. Patty was the one who recommended Dr. Schulman to me, and she practices in my area.

Patty has always talked about the importance of vision therapy for people with autism, ADHD, Sensory Processing Disorder, learning disabilities and other neurological disorders. Now I know why. In fact, Patty's book was published by the Optometric Extension Program Foundation, which should give you a clue as to the importance of vision in neurodevelopmental disorders.

Dr. Schulman believes that visual problems can affect cognitive, speech-language and social-emotional development, and she relates many cases in these chapters of children who showed great gains in social or language ability after beginning vision therapy. One child made eye contact for the first time, another spoke in full sentences for the first time.

However, only about a third of patients see immediate gains on the first visit, but many more see big gains after weekly vision therapy sessions. Dr. Schulman points out that,

"Most children do not outgrow delays in visual development without intervention."[26]

Understanding the Development of the Sensory System

To understand why children can see gains in these seemingly unrelated areas, you need to understand how the sensory system develops and how it is affected by primitive reflexes.

Gross-motor delays are common in children with neurodevelopmental disorders, especially if they skip or move too quickly through a developmental phase. I experienced this with my own two sons: my older son didn't walk until he was 20 months old, my younger son when he was 16 months. My older son cross-crawled for only a few weeks, and cross-crawling is imperative for wiring the brain for correct vision as it is the same ratio as an older child looking at his desk. Remember that vision is not seeing. Vision is what happens inside the brain once the eyes have seen.

Vision at the Top of the Hierarchy of Senses

There is a hierarchy of senses, and vision is at the top, meaning that other senses must develop first before proper vision occurs. As babies get older, a neurotypical child inhibits primitive reflexes that are necessary to integrate the senses and provide the ability to sit up straight, cross-crawl and walk. Dr. Schulman writes, "Vision develops according to a hierarchy, and vision development will be delayed by immature oral and motor development."[27]

Retention of these reflexes is common in children with

---

26. Lemer, Patricia S. (Ed.), *Envisioning a Bright Future: Interventions that Work for Children and Adults with Autism Spectrum Disorders.* Santa Ana, CA: OEP Foundation, Inc., 2008, 197.

27. Ibid, 23.

neurodevelopmental disorders, which is why they may appear, to the unknowing person, to be more clumsy and/or to have poor gross- and fine-motor skills, which can ultimately lead to poor social skills. She writes that, "Postural warps can mirror visual dysfunctions and asymmetries – either caused by or causing them."[28] It's fairly easy to spot a child, even a baby, with a developmental delay: they're typically the ones with poor posture.

Dr. Schulman also points out that, "Children who have poor oral motor skills such as sucking, blowing or swallowing ability often have convergence problems that can improve once the oral concerns have been addressed."[29] This is due to a poor rooting reflex, which causes a baby to turn its head and open its mouth in preparation for nursing. And what does a baby do when she's breastfeeding? She looks at her mom! This is how babies learn to focus their eyes.

Children with vision problems typically also have hypersensitive hearing, and now I know why. Dr. Schulman writes that, "Many patients rely heavily on their auditory systems because the visual systems are so inefficient and unreliable." Huh. So, correcting vision would reduce the stress load on the hearing system. Interesting!

These children typically also have acute senses of taste and smell, which makes them picky eaters. They "often prefer less typically used senses of taste and smell to gain information. They smell or taste inedible objects, and use touch instead of vision to gain information." I wonder if the same logic holds true: that if vision were corrected, these children might become less picky in their eating?

Factors Affecting Vision Development

Even though I've read a lot about developmental delays, primitive reflexes and neurodevelopmental disorders, Dr. Schulman pointed out some things that were interesting to me,

28. Ibid, 33.
29. Ibid, 35.

and of which I'd never heard or read, especially as it relates to vision. The most outstanding point is that, "Inadequate or inappropriate sensory stimulation and health problems, ranging from food allergies to ear infections and asthma can all disrupt vision development."[30]

She also writes that, "Risk factors for visual problems include frequent illness, particularly ear and strep infections, and their treatment with antibiotics."[31] I betcha very few pediatricians know about this risk, despite the fact that many of them hand out antibiotic prescriptions as if they were candy. Ugh.

Strabismus

Many children with neurodevelopmental disorders have an eye turn, called a "strabismus." An ophthalmologist would typically recommend surgery, but Dr. Schulman points out that, in many cases, this condition can be corrected with vision therapy. Besides, fixing the eye with surgery is only a cosmetic patch and does nothing to fix the incorrect vision that causes the strabismus. "It's not ...an 'eyeball' problem, but rather... a brain dysfunction."[32]

I urge you to seek out care from a behavioral / developmental optometrist as one of your first choices for therapy, as the vision correction he or she provides can head off some of the other sensory issues that these children have and potentially lead to better social interaction. Reading Patty's book and Dr. Schulman's chapters in it will give you a very clear understanding of how these practitioners use prisms, yoked prisms, colored lenses, visual arousal activities and more to improve vision.

30. Ibid, 27.
31. Ibid, 29.
32. Ibid, 208.

Look into Neurodevelopmental Movement

Neurodevelopmental movement is a great way to lower stress, improve sleep and integrate retained reflexes. It can optimize the brain and sensory processing for children with Sensory Processing Disorder, autism, PDD-NOS, ADHD, and learning disabilities.

When most people think of movements to help the brain, they may think of cross-pattern or crawling movements, but there are a large number of foundational brain-based movements from infancy that come before crawling that many SPD kids are missing. These missing neurodevelopmental movements can cause gaps in their ability to process their senses. Sonia Story of Move, Play, Thrive is an expert in the field, and she offers training in neurodevelopmental movement including Rhythmic Movement Training over the internet for your child.

The Masgutova Method, also known as Masgutova Neurosensorimotor Integration (MNRI), is renowned for reflex integration and is another form of neurodevelopmental movement. There are only a few therapists that have been trained in this method, but you can always purchase books and videos about the subject from the website www.masgutovamethod.com. Athena Oden's *Ready Bodies, Learning Minds* offers similar information, and I find her books easy for a parent to navigate and use.

Try Aquatic Therapy

Aquatic therapy is for children with developmental delays, gross motor delays and sensory issues, especially those concerning water. This can include kids with Sensory Processing Disorder, learning disabilities, ADHD, autism, PDD-NOS, speech delays, apraxia and dyspraxia.

This is terrific for reflex-integration as well. My friends Cindy Freedman and Ailene Tisser at Angelfish Therapy provide this to those in the NYC/Boston area and also offer

DVDs for those who want to learn how to do this at home. In addition, drowning is one of the leading causes of death for children with autism, and Cindy and Ailene teach you how to teach your child how to be safe around water.

My older son worked with Cindy Freedman for almost two years for "neuromuscular reeducation" while my younger son, whose retained reflexes weren't quite as severe, worked with another aquatic OT for four months. I realized my younger son had vestibular processing problems when he was a toddler because I would take him to mommy-and-me swimming classes; even though I was holding on to him firmly, he would say "I'm falling, I'm falling" when he wasn't.

This therapy wasn't cheap, and we had to pay out of pocket, but I strongly believe that this kind of intervention will pay off huge dividends in both sons' social skills, learning abilities, sports abilities (not that sports was the driver for receiving therapy), and, ultimately, happiness.

Get an Auditory Therapy Assessment

Many SPD kids have auditory processing problems, as evidenced by them crying and covering their ears when sounds are too loud, although some children are hyposensitive. A client of mine's son was so hypersensitive to sound that he couldn't go outside because the sound of bugs flying would upset him. For a child like this, auditory therapy is a must, although dealing with primitive-reflex integration and vision therapy first is a good idea. Often, SPD kids overcompensate with hearing because they have visual processing problems.

There are two kinds of auditory therapy that most parents will find: AIT (Auditory Integration Training), developed by Dr. Guy Berard, and the Tomatis method, although there are other therapies such as BioAcoustics, the Interactive Metronome and spinoffs of the Tomatis Method and Berard's AIT. For more information about any of these, I refer you to Patricia Lemer's *Envisioning a Bright Future: Interventions that Work for Children and Adults with Autism Spectrum Disorders,* which has an entire chapter discussing all of these methods.

The Tomatis Method uses an Electronic Ear. Three types of sounds are played through it to correct auditory processing problems: Mozart, Gregorian chants and mom's voice. By listening to these sounds while filtering out or in certain frequencies, the Electronic Ear trains parts of your child's ears to work together. Therapy is usually conducted for two sets of 15 days for two hours per day.

AIT is an intensive 10-day listening program. As I've established earlier in this book, a processing disorder is often caused by toxicity, but Dr. Bernard Rimland discovered two interesting points: 1) an auditory processing problem can be merely the result of a magnesium deficiency, and 2) removing the source of toxicity and/or correcting nutritional deficiencies can sometimes be enough to correct auditory processing problems.[33] Parents may find that their children sweat more during this intensive period, and that's actually a good thing because sweating is a great way for your child to detoxify! Just be sure to supplement with extra magnesium during the intensive.

Have Your Child Do Swimming and Taekwondo

Both swimming and taekwondo are beneficial to SPD kids because they can promote reflex integration; taekwondo, in particular, helps because children cross the midline. Although they are solo sports, they can both also instill a sense of confidence and accomplishment in your child.

Do Head-Tilting Exercises

Head-tilting exercises are a great way for you to stimulate your child's vestibular system, which, in a way, controls many of the other senses. To do this, have your child lie on the edge of a bed with his or her head hanging over the side; you can start with your child on his or her back, stomach or either side.

---

33. Ibid, 225.

Set a metronome to 60 beats per minute, then lift your child's head up as far as it can go to a count of eight, keeping time with the beat. Do this for three sets on each side.

Raising pH Levels

Increasing your child's pH level can help your with reversing sensory symptoms because doing so lowers your child's inflammation. A low, acidic pH can be associated with colds, the flu, viral infections, allergies, asthma, cancer and neurological disorders such as Sensory Processing Disorder. A low pH is especially dangerous to your child's mitochondria, which are responsible for energy production. I'll discuss mitochondria more later in the book.

A slightly alkaline body pH of 7.35–7.45 is optimal, although a pH between 7.0 and 7.45 is fine for detoxification. Buy pH test strips and check your child's saliva or urine regularly. The best time to test saliva is in the morning before your child has had any food or drink or two hours after they've eaten.

It's far easier to correct a too-alkaline pH rather than a too-acidic condition because we are constantly bombarded with acid-causing foods, stress and inflammation. The Standard American Diet (SAD) is very acidic because it's full of sugar, processed grains, starches, meats and dairy, all of which are acidic (sugar being the most acidic). SAD foods are typically low in alkaline foods such as sea vegetables, vegetables and sea salt.

The pH of most people is too acidic. Raising pH can help lower inflammation as well as make your child's body an inhospitable environment for pathogenic yeast, bacteria and parasites. The best way to increase your child's alkalinity is to have them:

- Eat more vegetables, especially sea vegetables.
- Get more minerals from animal organs, bone broth, vegetables and supplements.
- Use a sea/land salt with lots of trace minerals.

- Drink smoothies with barley grass juice powder, which is gluten-free.
- Drink the juice of a freshly squeezed lemon in water.
- Ingest a small amount of baking soda in water, although this tastes salty and may make them feel queasy for a little while. Adding lemon juice makes this more palatable.
- Eliminate sugar, the most inflammatory food.
- Reduce toxicity.
- Have your child take baths with one cup of baking soda and one cup of dead sea salts/magnesium chloride. Doing this creates magnesium bicarbonate, a powerful alkalizing and detoxifying agent, as Mark Sircus describes in *Sodium Bicarbonate – Full Medical Review.*

HEALING THE GUT

After lowering your child's stress levels, the next step is for you to heal your child's gut because healing the gut helps the rest of your child's body heal. Inflammation is lowered, more neurotransmitters are made, and the immune system is strengthened by healing the gut. We'll start by looking at your child's digestion to see if it can be improved, then we'll take a look at what your child is eating. As Hippocrates said so long ago, "Let food be your medicine, and let medicine be your food."

You'll want to give your child high-quality foods such as organic fruits and vegetables as well as pastured animal products; preparing foods properly ensure maximum nutrients for your child. Hopefully by now, you're not giving your child the inflammatory and toxic foods that I discussed in previous chapters such as GMOs foods and foods with additives such as artificial colors, flavors and preservatives.

It's likely that you'll need to implement a specific dietary protocol. A gluten-free, dairy-free diet is usually where most parents start, but given that your child may have yeast overgrowth or pathogenic infection, a gut-healing diet is likely in order.

Boosting Immunity by Improving Digestion

Roughly 70% of the immune system is in the gut, so it's important that the whole gastrointestinal system is performing optimally for your child's health to improve and symptoms to go away. In addition, most viruses, bacteria and parasites enter the body through the mouth.

Increase Stomach Acid

It's important that your child have enough stomach acid to be able to digest food properly. If your child failed the baking soda test mentioned earlier in the book, there are a few things you can do to increase the levels.

- Have your child drink a glass of water 20 minutes before a meal.
- Don't let your child drink water with a meal unless it's sparkling water, which is slightly acidic.
- Give your child a little raw apple cider vinegar in water before a meal.

Supplement with Digestive Enzymes

If your child's test showed that he or she has low levels of pancreatic enzymes, giving them digestive enzymes will help them digest their food better, leading to better nutritional absorption.

Increase Bile Production

Bile is necessary for the digestion of fats as well as for

raising the alkalinity of food after it leaves the stomach, thereby preparing it for further digestion in the small intestine. Hardened bile can clog the liver, gallbladder and ducts between each other as well as to the pancreas. You can stimulate bile production in your child by having them eat more bitter greens, raw beets and fenugreek seeds. This will help your child to digest fats better. Examples of bitter greens are asparagus, artichoke, dandelion greens, arugula and kale. In traditional Chinese restaurants there is usually some form of bitter vegetable served.

Limit Snacks

It's a very American thing to have snacks between meals; many other cultures don't even have a word for snack! The digestive tract needs a break between meals. If your child is constantly snacking, undigested food begins to putrefy, creating a breeding ground for pathogens. Between meals is when proteolytic enzymes come into play; their job is to digest protein casings from viruses, bacteria and cancer cells. If your child snacks a lot, these enzymes won't be able to do their job well. To limit snacks, be sure your child is getting enough protein and fat during each meal to fill them up.

Check the Poop

Your child should be pooping at least once a day, but chronic constipation is rampant in children these days. I don't recommend that children take fiber, enemas and laxatives because they can be addictive, making it hard to poop without them. In addition, for some children, adding fiber is liking adding hair to a clogged drain. For a great explanation of this, read *Fiber Menace: The Truth About the Leading Role of Fiber in Diet Failure, Constipation, Hemorrhoids, Irritable Bowel Syndrome, Ulcerative Colitis, Chron's Disease, and Colon Cancer* by Konstantin Monastyrsky. In the meantime, here are things you can do to keep things moving along:

- Have your child drink lots of water
- Have your child exercise
- Cut out gluten ("glue") and dairy (what Elmer's glue is made from – that's why it has a picture of a cow on it!)
- Give your child magnesium
- Give your child vitamin C
- Have your child drink green juice. My colon hydro-therapist calls it "soap" for the intestines. Speaking of which, colonics are a great way to help the body detoxify, but I'm hesitant to recommend giving them to a child.
- Get a squatty potty for your child. Putting the knees above the level of the hips helps gravity do its job better.

Eating High-Quality Foods

There's a famous saying, "You can pay the farmer now or pay the doctor later," and I truly believe it. Having your child avoid processed food, eat high-quality food that he or she isn't sensitive to, and eat more vegetables will do a lot to improve your child's health.

Another way to create health is to eat fresh-as-possible foods. Americans typically eat far more processed foods loaded with subsidized crops such as corn, soy, dairy and sugar than other cultures do. A Time photo-essay called "Hungry Planet: What the World Eats" shows that most other cultures eat far more fresh food and less processed food than Americans do.[1] Many times, processed foods contain preservatives, trans fats, sugar, artificial colors, antibiotics, growth hormones and, sometimes, even carcinogens. No wonder Americans have such high healthcare expenses!

---

1. http://time.com/8515/hungry-planet-what-the-world-eats/. Accessed September 3, 2014.

Eat Organic Foods

True, organic food costs more money up front, but as Benjamin Franklin is famously quoted as saying "A stitch in time saves nine." One of the best ways to create health is to eat organic foods. Pesticides used in non-organic foods have been linked time and again to diseases and disorders ranging from cancer to Parkinson's to autism and ADHD.[2]

There's a video on YouTube of a girl's science experiment with organic versus non-organic sweet potatoes that you and your child can do at home to convince yourselves of the dangers of eating non-organic foods.[3] In three weeks, the organic sweet potato is full of leafy green vines; the non-organic one has none because it's been sprayed with "bud nip," also used on blueberries, carrots and onions, to prevent plants from budding; it's been linked to cancer.

Yes, organic foods cost more, but consider that the typical American family pays less than half of what other cultures do because so many of our unhealthy crops are subsidized such as sugar, corn, wheat, soy and canola.[4] Joel Salatin, founder of Polyface Farms and author of *Folks, This Ain't Normal: A Farmer's Advice for Happier Hens, Healthier People and a Better World,* says "If you think the price of organic food is expensive, have you priced cancer lately?"

It can be expensive to have your child eat as many organic foods as possible, so I recommend you use the Environmental Working Group's Shopper's Guide to Pesticides in Produce to know which non-organic produce is safest.[5] The EWG lists the Clean 15, the 15 safest non-organic fruits and vegetables as:

---

2. Vogt, R., et al, Cancer and non-cancer health effects from food contaminant exposures for children and adults in California: a risk assessment, *Environ Health.* 2012 Nov 9;11:83.
3. https://www.youtube.com/watch?v=exBEFCiWyW0. Accessed September 9, 2014.
4. http://farm.ewg.org/region.php. Accessed September 3, 2014.
5. http://www.ewg.org/foodnews/. Accessed September 3, 2014.

- Avocados
- Sweet corn
- Pineapples
- Cabbage
- Sweet peas (frozen)
- Onions
- Asparagus
- Mangoes
- Papayas
- Kiwi
- Eggplant
- Grapefruit
- Cantaloupe (domestic)
- Cauliflower
- Sweet potatoes

The EWG also has a list of the Dirty Dozen, 12+ foods that should *always* be organic because they are so heavily sprayed with pesticides, which are known to cause neurodevelopmental damage.

- Apples
- Strawberries
- Grapes
- Celery
- Peaches
- Spinach
- Sweet bell peppers
- Nectarines (imported)
- Cucumbers
- Cherry tomatoes
- Snap peas (imported)
- Potatoes
- Hot peppers
- Blueberries (domestic)
- Any leafy green

You can also join a CSA (Community Supported Agriculture) and support your local, organic farmers. By buying a share in a CSA farm, you're sharing the risks and rewards. If the farm has a great year, your share buys a bumper crop; if the weather is bad and/or pests destroy the crops, your share buys very little. It's important that we support local farms so that all of our food doesn't wind up under the control of Big Ag.

Eat Pastured Meats, Dairy and Eggs

I recommend that your child eat pastured, pasture-raised or grass-fed eggs, chickens, beef and lamb because these animals are eating what nature intended them to eat and are typically free of antibiotics, growth hormones, GMOs and inflammatory foods like corn and soy. They also have higher levels of beneficial fatty acids, such as conjugated linoleic acid (CLA) in grass-fed beef, butter and other dairy products, in comparison to feed-lot animals. In my opinion, feed-lot animals are raised inhumanely, as they are typically confined to pens so small that they can't even turn around. These animals are under severe stress, and they get sick a lot, which is why they are given high doses of antibiotics. Even if your meats and eggs are organic, they are likely just eating organic corn and soy, yet still confined to an inhumane pen.

When it comes to eggs, don't be misled by the term "cage free"; it's a meaningless term. Instead, look for the "Certified Humane" label on your eggs. Unless they're from your local farmer, pasture-raised eggs are typically certified humane.

Have you ever compared the yolk of a pasture-raised egg to a typical grocery store egg? The yolk of the pasture-raised egg is a beautiful dark orange because the chickens are eating bugs, as they should be, which give them proper nutrients. Grocery store eggs are an anemic, pale yellow. Raising chickens in the backyard is a fairly easy thing to do, and I have quite a few friends that are doing so! It makes me happy to see people taking food quality back into their own hands.

Preparing Food Properly

Modern, convenience foods do nothing for our health. I used to eat them, too, but after experiencing first-hand how eating real food, not just food-like products, has improved the health of my children and my clients' children, I am now a big fan of eating traditionally prepared foods. A great place to learn about them is *Nourishing Traditions: The Cookbook that Challenges Politically Correct Nutrition and the Diet Dictocrats* by Sally Fallon and Mary Enig of the Weston A. Price Foundation. Think about it: people were a whole lot healthier before the introduction of processed foods and the introduction of refrigeration, pasteurization and chemical preservatives.

Eat Whole Foods

I recommend that your child eat whole foods, not foods "made with whole foods." If they're eating cereals, switch to gluten-free oat groats, amaranth or buckwheat kasha. You'll find these in the bulk foods section of Whole Foods or other health-food stores. For lunch and dinner, you can make your own French fries from potatoes, sweet potatoes, beets, rutabagas, and turnips, or make a quinoa tabouli, for example. Once you get out of processed-food land, you'll discover that there is a whole world of other foods to eat! Try challenging yourself next time you go the market to buy and cook a whole food that your child hasn't eaten before like jicama, burdock or daikon radish.

You'll feel better feeding your SPD child real, homemade, whole, nutritious foods. Now that you know what problems the Standard American Diet creates for your child, it's hard to let them have any kind of non-organic, genetically modified, gluten- and dairy-filled foods. You can't unknow this!

In addition to removing sugar, high fructose corn syrup, vegetable oils, trans fats and processed grains, you'll also want to get rid of low-fat/non-fat foods, GMOs, artificial colors, artificial flavors, preservatives, artificial sweeteners and flavor enhancers.

Soak Grains, Legumes, Nuts and Seeds

You'll want to soak all legumes, nuts, seeds and grains, including brown rice, for at least eight hours to remove phytic acid, a potent digestive inhibitor. The easiest thing is to use a 1/2 gallon Mason jar with a special sprouting lid that lets you drain off the water. These foods can be soaked and "sprouted" for up to three days, but if you're going to do it for that long, you need to be sure to rinse and drain every eight hours.

After sprouting nuts and seeds, you'll want to put them in a dehydrator to remove the water; otherwise, they'll get moldy. I recommend doing this to nuts and seeds in large batches, then freezing after dehydrated.

Throw Out Your Microwave

Your child's health is compromised when eating microwaved food. Not only do microwaves lower the nutritional value of food[6], but they also leach plastics into the food itself. In addition, microwaves also change the physical structure of both food and water, so don't even microwave water.[7]

Do you know that microwaves are banned in Russia because of how damaging they are to health? The Russians discovered that carcinogens are made from microwaving all different kinds of food. I freaked when I read about this because I had been eating Lean Cuisines and Healthy Choice microwavable meals for years thinking I was healthy. Not.

---

6. Lee L. "Health effects of microwave radiation-microwave ovens," *Lancet* December 9, 1989 (article)
7. http://articles.mercola.com/sites/articles/archive/2010/05/18/microwave-hazards.aspx. Accessed September 9, 2014.

Some microwaves may actually leak their radiation. An easy way to check this is to put your cell phone into the microwave. Don't turn the microwave on, of course! Call your cell phone from your land line. If it rings while in the microwave, this means that your microwave isn't sealed well and allows microwaves, on which your cell phone operates, in and out. Even standing one foot away from your microwave while it's on can expose you to over 400 milliGauss of radiation; a dose of only four milliGauss has been linked to leukemia.[8]

Here's what I do to reheat food: I put a small amount of water, maybe a tablespoon or more, into a small pan, put the food in, put the lid on and reheat on the stove. You can use a toaster oven, too, to reheat bready things. Yes, this process takes longer, but it's a necessary adjustment. Your child's health is more important than the convenience of microwaving your food and water.

Overcoming Gut Dysbiosis

Gut dysbiosis is an imbalance of beneficial bacteria and yeast in the intestines versus pathogenic yeast, bacteria, viruses and parasites. It is a major factor in chronic illnesses today, including Sensory Processing Disorder. Given that most of these children have systemic *Candida* overgrowth and that antifungal drugs against it have only limited effectiveness, it makes sense to look into what you can do at home to stem the dysbiosis.

In a nutshell, here are the basic steps to healing gut dysbiosis:

- Eliminate unfermented dairy, gluten, sugar and refined foods. In addition, different diets have different protocols for removing grains and starches.
- Take probiotics.

---

8. Ibid.

- Eat fermented foods, which contain naturally occurring probiotics.
- Eat mineral-rich foods because pathogens use them up.
- Using anti-microbial herbs and foods such as oregano, rosemary, thyme, turmeric, garlic, basil and coconut oil.
- Eat pastured and organic, non-GMO foods.

These are the basics, but they may not be enough. Instead, you may need to implement a gut-healing diet, which I'll go over later in this chapter.

Many parents are discovering that cutting out gluten and dairy can have profound benefits on reversing their child's sensory issues and health issues, and there's a good chance that if you did the elimination diet for your SPD child, you found out he or she was sensitive to both of these foods. One of the reasons that removing gluten and dairy can be so helpful to your child's health is that both of these foods are constipating, meaning that toxins that should be pooped out aren't. Both of these foods, eaten in the typical Standard American Diet, also contribute to gut dysbiosis. Remember that gluten has the word "glue" in it and that Elmer's glue has a picture of a cow on it. It's made from milk, and that milk becomes glue in your child's intestine.

In addition, gluten and casein (the protein found in dairy) can escape the intestines of people with leaky guts. When they reach the brain, they can activate the same receptors as morphine and heroin, making your child who's just eaten macaroni and cheese seem as if they are on drugs, acting very spacey and unfocused. Thus, removing gluten and dairy foods can improve your child's attention. A gluten-free, casein-free diet helps most children with SPD.

Removing gluten and dairy from your child's diet can be overwhelming because those foods are likely 90% of their diets. A good place to start is *The Kid-Friendly ADHD and Autism Cookbook: The Ultimate Guide to the Gluten-Free, Casein-Free Diet* by Pamela Compart and Dana Laake. I found this to be an enormously helpful resource not only in providing gluten-free, casein-free recipes but also in giving pertinent information about food allergies and their effect.

Remove Dairy

Taking dairy out of your child's diet is challenging, but there is a whole world of substitutes out there: almond milk, coconut milk, hemp milk, rice milk. I don't recommend soy milk because it is unfermented soy, which is damaging to the thyroid. If you buy store-bought dairy alternatives, be sure they don't have carrageenan in them, which is a potential carcinogen; most dairy alternatives contain this harmful ingredient. If you have the time, I recommend making homemade nut or coconut milks, which involves blending the nuts or coconut flakes in water, then straining off the meat. You can use the leftovers for cooking other items.

If you or your pediatrician are worried about where your child gets his or her calcium, just remember to get it from where the cows do: leafy greens such as spinach. Broccoli, dried figs, sesame seeds and sardines are other excellent sources of calcium.

It was after my older son had a severe asthma attack and was prescribed a nebulizer, steroids and an inhaler when he was four years old that I took him to my naturopath for the first time. He immediately took my son off dairy. I was buying seven or eight six-packs of Pediasure® a week in those days because, by this time, both my sons had growth and developmental issues; they were also both on Prevacid® for their acid reflux. One of the first things I did, with the naturopath's feedback, was to make a dairy-free "homemade Pediasure®". If Pediasure® was the stopgap I used before, then "homemade Pediasure®" would be my new stopgap (see Recipes).

Voila, after removing dairy, his acid reflux cleared almost immediately, and I was able to stop giving them Prevacid®, which I now know is so damaging to health. My son hasn't had an asthma attack in the five years since.

If your child is prone to ear infections, one of the easiest ways to help prevent them is to remove dairy from your child's diet. That's because dairy, in an unfermented form, feeds gut pathogens and is mucous-forming.

I was completely thrilled to have both of my sons off of Prevacid® and my older son asthma-free! However, neither their multiple pediatricians, their allergist nor their gastroenterologist ever suggested removing dairy from their diets. That's because doctors are taught next to nothing about nutrition in medical school.

Remove Gluten

A whole host of publications have come out recently that argue against gluten in the diet (*Grain Brain*, *Wheat Belly* and "The Dark Side of Wheat"), mainly because the gluten we eat today, which comes mainly in the form of wheat, although it is also found in barley, rye and non-gluten-free oats, is not the same as what our grandparents ate. Wheat has been hybridized and genetically manipulated to the extent that our bodies recognize it as foreign and unfriendly. In fact, recently there was an online "Gluten Summit," in which celiac researchers, functional-medicine doctors and holistic nutritionists collectively agreed that gluten should be removed from most, if not all, of our diets.

As more and more people discover that their allergies, asthma, autoimmune diseases and neurodevelopmental disorders are exacerbated by food allergies and intolerances, these people discover that removing allergenic foods, such as gluten, from their diets makes them feel better. Removing gluten from your child's diet can relieve him or her from a lot of symptoms that you might typically give an over-the-counter medication for such as bloating, headaches, constipation, diarrhea, inability to focus, fatigue and joint pain. Beware of hidden sources of gluten, such as those found in salad dressings, soups, puddings, processed meats and ice cream.

I don't recommend that you replace all of your gluten-filled foods with their gluten-free counterparts. Doing so will get you a lot of gluten-free junk food. Typically, these pancakes, cookies, waffles and breads are loaded with corn and potato starch as dough softeners, and adding more of these high-glycemic starches to your diet can adversely affect your child's blood sugar.

Instead, I recommend adding in gluten-free whole foods into your child's diet: brown rice, wild rice, buckwheat, millet, amaranth, quinoa, teff, sorghum, non-GMO corn and potatoes are great starting points. If you're baking, my favorite grain-based gluten-free flour is sorghum, or you could try non-grain flours made from coconuts or nuts.

Add in Probiotics

Refrigerated probiotics typically have more live cultures in them unless they're listed as "shelf stable." I recommend that you start your child on a high-quality, multi-strain probiotic at a small dose, then work up to larger doses to avoid symptoms of pathogen die-off such as:

- Nausea
- Headache, fatigue, dizziness
- Swollen glands
- Bloating, gas, constipation or diarrhea
- Increased joint or muscle pain
- Elevated heart rate
- Chills, cold feeling in your extremities
- Body itchiness, hives or rashes
- Sweating
- Fever
- Skin breakouts
- Recurring vaginal infections, prostate infections and sinus infections

Add in Fermented Foods

Unpasteurized fermented foods are a great source of naturally occurring probiotics, and they can contain much higher levels of probiotics than supplements do. Giving your child foods such as kim chi, sauerkraut, fermented pickles, fermented carrots and fermented beets is an easy way to get loads of probiotics into them. Just make sure they are the refrigerated kind; not the kind sitting on the shelf brined in vinegar. These foods are actually very easy to make at home, just as our grandparents and ancestors did for thousands of years.

Fermented foods are contraindicated for people who are sensitive to histamines, and you'll need to start your child slowly on these foods as well, while watching for signs of die-off.

Applying a Gut-Healing Diet

I know it's difficult to implement one of these gut-healing diets because I have tried them all, and implementing them is not something you can do overnight. My best advice is to gear up for it by finding recipes that work for you and your family before you decide to pull the plug on everything else. Otherwise, your child is going to be pretty hungry for a while and wonder, "What is there to eat?"

In addition, your child may do well on one of these diets for a while but then hit a plateau in which there seems to be no more improvement in health. At that point, you might want to switch to another gut-healing diet. Remember, every child is different, so what works for one won't always work for your child.

If your child does hit a plateau, I suggest you also look into some of the hidden food sensitivities discussed earlier in the book such as phenols, histamines, glutamates and oxalates. I highly recommend Julie Matthews' book, *Nourishing Hope for Autism: Nutrition and Diet Guide for Healing Children: ADHD, Autism, Learning and Developmental Delays*, for ferreting out these issues.

I recommend that you start with one of the following gut-healing diets for a minimum of three months, then switch if you don't see any gains. There's a good chance that your child shows improvement immediately upon starting one of these diets, or at least within a few days. Stick with the diet, and if there's an infraction, just do like you do when you fall off a bike: get back on it and keep going. Remember, it takes time to heal the gut, so in many cases your child may need to be on one of these diets for up to two years to allow the gut to heal.

These diets require your full commitment, and you have to cook almost all of your food, although you might luck out like I did and found some healthfully prepared foods that list the ingredients so you know what to avoid.

There is a large and growing number of people who are interested in recovering themselves or their children, so I encourage you to find them in groups on Facebook or to do Google searches for recipes and blogs. It's an all-consuming lifestyle for a while, but isn't it worth it for your child to heal?

Anti-Candida Diet

Personally, I don't recommend this diet because it's way too restrictive, so I'm not going to get into it here. In this diet, you have to eliminate all sugars, starches, grains, fruits, dairy, vinegars and alcohols. With that said, however, the following gut-healing diets do omit these foods in varying combinations.

Body Ecology Diet

The Body Ecology Diet is a gut-healing diet that I highly recommend. To me, it is the most comprehensive approach to healing the gut, and therefore the body, because Donna Gates, its developer, addresses hormonal balances of the adrenals and thyroid; as far as I know, hers is the only gut-healing diet that does. She emphasizes the use of sea vegetables to heal the thyroid and adrenals. All in all, it's a very well-thought-out and comprehensive diet that offers health-promoting principles for everyone.

Her book, *The Body Ecology Diet: Recovering Your Health and Rebuilding Your Immunity*, is very helpful at explaining gut dysbiosis and how to treat it. The protocol she offers will put you at odds with the Standard American Diet (SAD), but it works. The SAD contains too many processed, refined, sweetened and antibiotic-laden foods and can lead to gut dysbiosis. In contrast, the Body Ecology Diet (BED) eliminates gluten, dairy, sugars and most fruits (although fruit can be added in later) because they all feed yeast and pathogens. BED also teaches the principles of 80/20, uniqueness, food combining, eating fermented foods, acid/alkaline and step by step.

An alkaline diet is more healthful as it is more vegetable-based whereas the SAD is a very acidic diet, which can leave your child open to infectious invasion. An overly acidic diet (sugars, processed foods, meats, grains, dairy) creates an acidic environment in the body, making it more hospitable to pathogens like viruses, strep, *Clostridium*, Lyme disease infections, other pathogenic bacteria, *Candida* and other yeast, and parasites. Eating a more alkaline diet (vegetables and sea vegetables) alkalizes the diet and helps prevent infections.

If you think about it, before the invention of refrigeration, all foods that our great-grandparents ate were fresh, preserved with salt (real salt, not the processed white stuff we find today) or preserved with fermentation. These are truly health-promoting foods! That's why the subtitle of this book is "Changing the Way the World Eats with Probiotic Nutrition."

I won't say it's an easy diet to follow, mostly because of the food-combining principle. You can have gluten-free grains on the diet, just not with protein, which is a nice highlight for people out there who feel better eating grains or those who need more carbohydrate-rich diets like children and athletes. To this end, Donna also includes Peter D'Adamo's Blood Type theory in the diet. However, food combining makes it a bit more challenging about when to eat things like olives, avocados, nuts, etc. If you're eating out, it's best to think Paleo-type foods, minus the nuts and fruit.

Paleo Diet

The Paleo, or primal, diet is often called the "caveman" diet because it's based on the idea of eating the fresh, unprocessed foods that a caveman would've eaten. There is a common misconception that the Paleo diet is very meat-centric. I disagree with this viewpoint. In all diets, including the Paleo diet, I recommend that your child use meat as a condiment and load up on the vegetables. The Paleo diet is the one used by Dr. Terry Wahls to recover herself from secondary progressive multiple sclerosis.

The Paleo diet excludes all legumes – peanuts, beans, lentils and peas – as well as grains, starches, processed foods and sugar; however, sweet potatoes and some starchy vegetables are allowed. A true Paleo diet has very little honey and fruits, as well, although the internet is rife with Paleo dessert recipes.

It is easy for your child to become too acidic on this diet if they don't eat enough broth, animal organs, vegetables and sea salt. Be sure to check their pH occasionally when following this diet. You can also correct pH by having your child supplement with baking soda, lemon juice and other items listed in the section, "Raising pH Levels."

Another drawback of this diet is that being on it can lead to high levels of oxalates that feed gut pathogens, thereby compounding the problem of gut dysbiosis. To avoid this problem, don't go nuts with the nuts because nuts and seeds are high in oxalates. If you're making bready foods such as waffles, muffins and pancakes for your child, lean more towards using coconut flour, which is a low-oxalate food. Be very careful when doing this, though, because you can't just substitute coconut flour for any other flour; it's too absorptive. Instead, find recipes made specifically for coconut flour. And don't be shocked by the amount of eggs and oil that you'll need to add to the recipe to keep from being too dry.

Specific Carbohydrate Diet / Gut And Psychology Syndrome Diet

The Specific Carbohydrate Diet (SCD) was developed by Elaine Gottschall as a way to heal her daughter of ulcerative colitis, which is a painful and bloody disorder. She discovered that her daughter's health improved when she stopped eating grains, sugars and starches, even though the girl's doctor insisted that food had nothing to do with the issue. In later years, as researchers discovered that many other chronic diseases and disorders have a gut-disorder component, SCD was used for conditions as seemingly different as asthma, allergies, lupus, autism, ADHD and even mood disorders.

With SCD, all grains and starches are eliminated. Fruit and honey are allowed because they are mono-saccharides and are digested quickly and don't lead to fermentation in the gut. Have you ever made bread at home? If so, you know that you need to add sugar to the yeast and dough to make the dough rise. What causes the dough to rise is the process of fermentation, which is the yeast digesting the sugar and releasing carbon dioxide, a gas. As the gas is made, it expands and causes the dough rise. The same thing happens in your child's gut when foods ferment, and this can lead to painful bloating before the gas is released from the body.

Many parents start with SCD because not only can their child have fruit and honey, but also fermented dairy such as homemade yogurt, kefir and aged cheeses, if tolerated. Aged cheeses include cheddar, Parmesan, asiago, Brie, Camembert, and blue. Store-bought yogurt and kefir are not allowed because they still have residual sugar as well as potential added sugar and fillers and they haven't been fermented for long enough.

In addition, nuts, navy beans, baby lima beans, peas and any kind of lentil are also allowed, which is why this diet is called the "Specific" Carbohydrate Diet; only specific carbohydrates are allowed. For parents following the diet, you'll feel less restricted by the diet knowing that occasional dry wine and dry liquor are allowed.

Dr. Natasha Campbell-McBride updated the SCD to what she calls the GAPS diet: Gut And Psychology Syndrome. The GAPS diet is essentially the SCD, but with more emphasis on the healing properties of bone broth, fats, fermented foods and juicing. Dr. Campbell-McBride, or Dr. Natasha as some people call her, recovered her son from autism with the GAPS diet. The GAPS diet has an introductory period where only a limited amount of foods are eaten to begin with to allow the gut to heal. Foods are then slowly added in to check for reactions. If you've done an elimination diet for your child, you may be able to skip this step as many parents have done or come back to it when the timing is better for your child's schedule, such as during the summer.

The SCD and GAPS diet are not low-fat diets at all, which is a real positive for controlling blood-sugar swings. Fats are extremely healing, despite what we've been taught to believe. They are necessary for the activation of the fat-soluble vitamins: vitamin A, vitamin D, vitamin E and vitamin K, and often contain them. In addition, because fruits, vegetables and certain legumes are the only sources of carbohydrates, the missing calories will need to be replaced with fat calories.

Both the SCD and GAPS diets recommend that you cook fruits and vegetables well to lower the amount of fiber in your child's gut; raw fruits and vegetables aren't allowed unless they're juice. This is the opposite of the advice that we're commonly given, but think about it: if you have a drain that's clogged with hair, do you add more hair to unclog it? No, you eliminate the hair and add something that will lubricate the hair and get it to flow through the pipes. The same can be said about adding fiber to the gut of an SPD child, who likely has chronic constipation/diarrhea. An interesting take on this subject is in Konstantin Monastyrsky's *Fiber Menace: The Truth About the Leading Role of Fiber in Diet Failure, Constipation, Hemorrhoids, Irritable Bowel Syndrome, Ulcerative Colitis, Chron's Disease, and Colon Cancer* as well as his website, www.gutsense.org.

The fruit, vegetables, lentils, peas and beans allowed on these diets can easily fill little tummies quickly, so be sure to give your child more fats from foods such as avocados, nuts and seeds to increase calorie density. Some children experience a slowdown in weight gain on these diets because they're not getting enough carbohydrates; some children don't. A low-carbohydrate diet can compound the adrenal problems that your child likely already has. Just remember that fruits, vegetables, lentils, peas and beans are the sources of carbohydrates in these diets.

As with the Paleo diet, it's easy for your child to become too acidic or consume too many oxalates with SCD and GAPS.

Case Study: Healing Eczema with the GAPS Diet

My sons had eczema for many years since they were born when they were younger. It has ranged from cradle cap (did you know that was a form of eczema?) to itchy bumps in the creases of the knees and elbows to full-blown bloody red rashes on the arms and legs.

The standard advice from our pediatricians was to "put a little cortisone cream on it." I did try that a few times at first with my older son, but I quickly grew worried about the effects of it on his already-poor immune system. Cortisone cream is a steroid, and steroids suppress the immune system. Not only that, but suppressing eczema with cortisone cream can lead to asthma because it drives the disease process deeper. Sure enough, after four years of using cortisone cream for my older son's eczema, he developed severe asthma and had to use a nebulizer, Xopenex and inhaled and liquid steroids.

Most times, we just put up with the itchiness, but a few winters ago, my older son's eczema was the worst I had ever seen. There was an itchy, red rash all over his thighs and horrible itchy bumps all around his elbow creases. He had scratched the bumps so much that they were constantly bleeding, and bathing or showering became a nightmare for him because the soap would sting. Here's what it looked like:

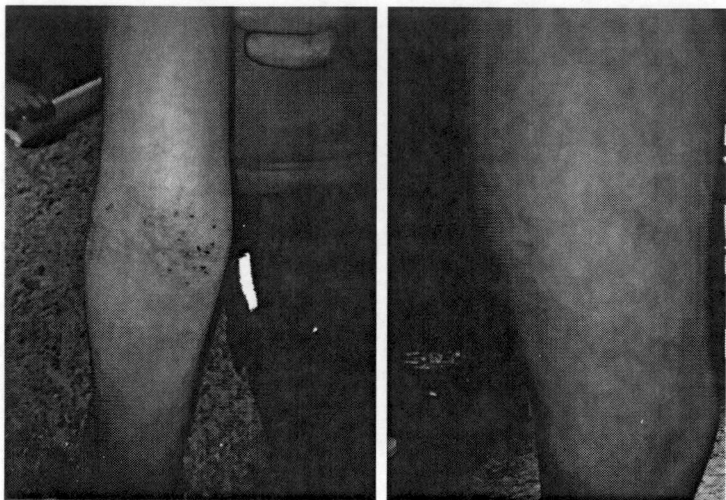

We began the full GAPS diet in the dead of winter. We had been on it for two weeks when my older son had one of the gluten-free, dairy-free, chocolate cupcakes that I had left in the nurse's office at school for school birthday parties. Here are pictures of the welts that appeared on him. The shininess is due to the anti-itch salve I had put on him.

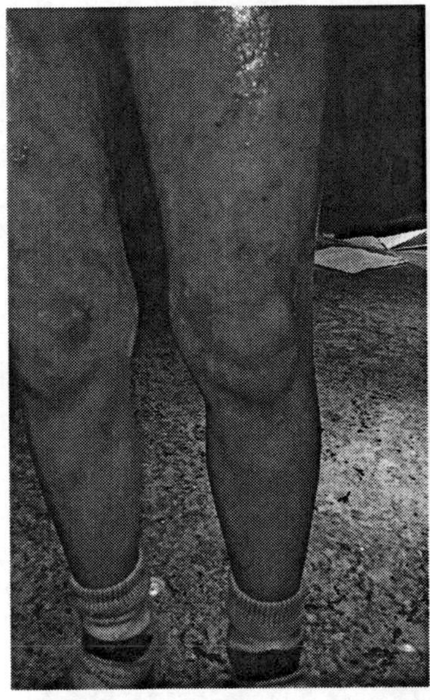

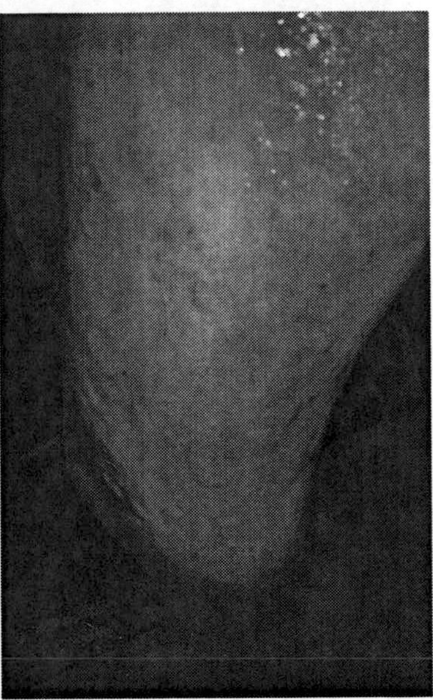

This kind of reaction was proof to me that the diet was working. The diet is so clean and healing that it unmasked unknown food sensitivities such as the chocolate, gluten-free grains, gluten-free starches and Rapidura sugar that I had used to make the chocolate cupcakes.

Just so you know, I didn't give him Benadryl®. Knowing what I know now about how pharmaceuticals poison pathways and the liver to alleviate symptoms (that's why there are side effects), I had tossed all the kids' medicines, including Benadryl®, Tylenol® and Motrin®. So what did I use to calm the inflammation? Cod liver oil and vitamin C, as they are both anti-inflammatory. They worked like a charm, eliminating the welts within 30 minutes. Now, why can't pediatricians recommend things like this that are not harmful and are actually quite helpful? Because they just don't know. They likely don't have time to research these issues independently. Pharmaceutical companies provide most of the education and training to doctors in medical school and in their practices, and what incentive do they have in promoting something natural that can't be patented? Zero.

His eczema slowly improved. Here's what it looked like after being on the GAPS diet for seven weeks:

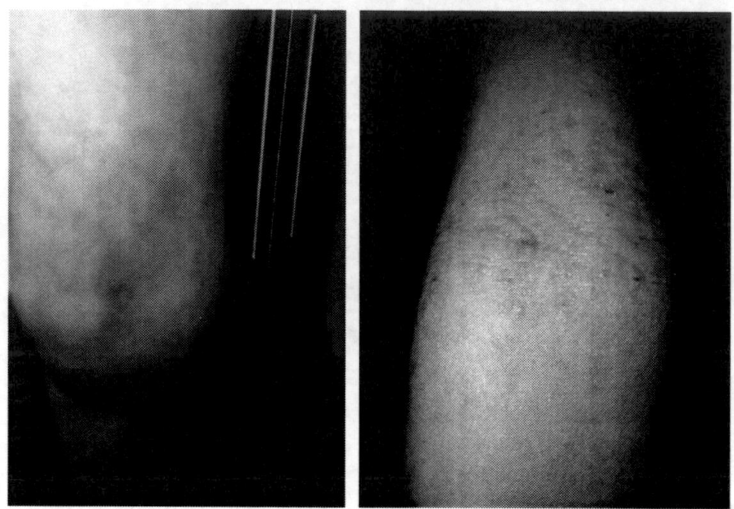

And here's what it looks like after almost five months on the diet:

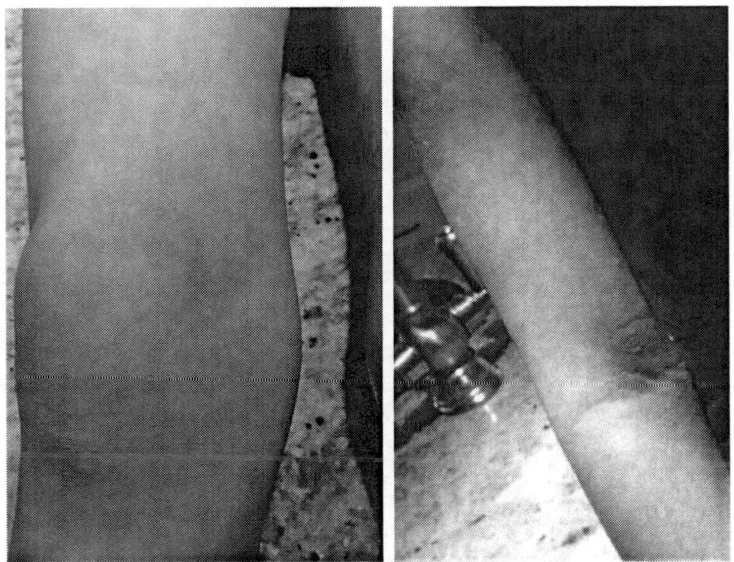

The eczema is completely gone from his arms and legs. He has been eczema-free ever since.

REMOVING TOXICITY

After reading about the causes of Sensory Processing Disorder, you should realize what a major role toxicity plays in damaging the neurodevelopment of our children. Not only are children born with unprecedented levels of heavy metals, pesticides, carcinogens and endocrine disruptors, but they are continually exposed to them on a daily basis.

Getting Rid of Toxicity Sources

I recommend removing the daily sources of exposure first, as these cause continuous stress to your child's body. It takes time, effort and money to replace them, but you'll find that every little tweak helps to weigh the balance of health in your child's favor. As I've said before, there's no one silver bullet that created this problem, and there's no one silver bullet that will undo it. Recovering your child's health is a marathon, not a sprint.

Clean Your Water

You might not know that there are a lot of potential hazards in your local drinking water. The Environmental

Working Group recently published a report, "Water Treatment Contaminants: Toxic Trash in Drinking Water,"[1] which found "probable human carcinogens" in every single water system they tested. They tested 201 municipal systems in 43 states.

Local water is typically fluoridated (fluoride is a known neurotoxin) and chlorinated, leading to extremely toxic disinfection byproducts (DBPs).[2] Pharmaceuticals, heavy metals, pesticides and more have been found in many water systems.

Even if your city water passes with flying colors, the local water board might not be testing for all toxins. In addition, even if the water is clean, many towns and cities have old, lead pipes that leach into the drinking water. Chicago, in particular, has found high levels of lead in its water. This article from the *Chicago Tribune* admits that "Current sampling methods may not be detecting all the lead in Chicago tap water."[3]

I recommend a reverse-osmosis (RO) water filtration system for your drinking and cooking water. It takes out all the heavy metals, chlorine, fluoride, everything. The problem is that this system is installed at your kitchen sink, so you won't be able to bathe and wash your clothes with this water. For that, you need to get a whole-house filter. It's not an RO system, but it does remove most fluoride and chlorine. Most people don't know that what goes on you, goes in you, which is why transdermal patches work so well; it only takes 26 seconds for something on the skin to be absorbed into the bloodstream. Even worse, toxins absorbed this way bypass the liver, leading to increased toxicity.

---

1. http://www.ewg.org/research/water-treatment-contaminants. Accessed August 28, 2014.
2. Ibid.
3. Eng, Monica. "Chicago water sampling shows high levels of lead", *Chicago Tribune*, January 31, 2012.

Clean Your Air

Newer fabric-covered furniture and mattresses typically are coated with neurotoxic flame retardants, which off-gas into the air. Paint often contains volatile organic compounds that off-gas, while new carpet and plywood-based, Ikea-ish furniture typically contain formaldehyde that off-gasses into your home. A HEPA filter is a great first step to removing toxins from the air, and NASA has published a list of common household plants that they discovered do an excellent job of purifying indoor air. Spider plants, dracaena ("cornstalk plant"), philodendrons, Gerber daisies, rubber plants and mother-in-law's tongue are all great choices for cleaning your air.

Clean with Non-Toxic Products

In the United States, it's not required that individual ingredients be listed in cleaning products for proprietary reasons. Luckily for us, the Environmental Working Group (EWG) tested common household cleaning products such as dishwasher detergent, laundry detergent, window cleaner and floor cleaner. Most products sold today are toxic. Don't assume, as I once did, that if it's sold in a store, it must be safe. It's very likely not.

The EWG put together a Cleaners database (www.ewg.org/guides/cleaners) in which you can check 2,000 different cleaning products for toxicity. If your product isn't listed in here, I would use a similar product with an "A" rating. What was shocking to me is that even products that are from seemingly non-toxic brands may not be. Don't just assume that if you have a Seventh Generation or Mrs. Meyers product that it's safe. You need to check each product individually. In addition, be sure to check back occasionally, as manufacturers are constantly rejiggering their formulas to manage their raw material supply and cost of production.

White vinegar mixed with water (I use a 1:2 ratio) is great for cleaning vegetables and countertops, as vinegar is anti-microbial. Baking soda and salt are also great non-toxic bases for cleaning; they are also anti-microbial. Many essential oils such as tea tree, lemon and lavender oils are safe and effective for cleaning when diluted in water, plus they smell great!

Check the Safety of Personal-Care Products

Most personal-care products in a typical grocery store or drugstore are loaded with toxic ingredients such as parabens, phthalates, mercury, lead, carcinogens, endocrine disruptors and neurotoxins. Again, don't assume that if it's sold, it must be safe. This applies to products such as shampoo, soaps, lotions, toothpaste, deodorants, cosmetics, hair dye and even baby-care products.

To check your cosmetics and personal-care products for toxic ingredients, use the Environmental Working Group's Skin Deep Cosmetics database at www.ewg.org/skindeep. If your particular product isn't listed, search the individual ingredients. I recommend using products with a 0, 1 or 2 safety rating. Don't fall for the misleading word "natural"; there's no official definition of what that is, and I've seen plenty of products boasting to be natural that are far from it.

My naturopath told me a long time ago that I should never put anything on my skin that I wouldn't put in my mouth. These days, we use coconut-oil based soaps, coconut oil, sesame oil or shea butter instead of lotion and fluoride-free, sodium-laureth-sulfate-free toothpastes.

Check the Safety of Toys and Clothes

Children are exposed to toxins even in their toys, books and games. An example of this was seen a few years ago when many popular Thomas the Tank Engine toys were recalled due to the high levels of lead in the paint, as they were made in China where there is little concern for safety. You can check for lead levels by using a home-based test kit that you can find online. One of my favorite places to learn about toy safety and toxicity is HealthyStuff.org. GreenToys.com is a good source to find toys that are free of BPA, PVC, phthalates and coatings.

Other children's toys to avoid are:

- Faux-leather goods (which contain lead)
- Cheap jewelry (which can contain lead, arsenic and cadmium)
- Some art supplies (which may contain lead, carcinogens and volatile organic compounds)

Avoid Synthetic Fragrances

Avoid using drier sheets and other scented products, even perfume. Artificial scents are typically endocrine disruptors, and they can also be neurotoxic. They are particularly dangerous for someone with asthma or other respiratory illnesses. A good start is to avoid products with added fragrances; look for "fragrance free" or "free and clear" on the label, but you still need to check the safety rating of these products, too. If you want things to smell nice, use essential oils in your laundry and use them in a diffuser to freshen up your air.

Use Non-Toxic Cookware and Dining Ware

You'll want to replace as much plastic as you can with glass to avoid exposure to phthalates from the plastics themselves. I use glass containers with plastic lids for storing my food, but I make sure that the lid doesn't touch the food and that the food isn't hot when I put the lid on. Ceramic dinnerware can contain very high amounts of heavy metals like lead and tin (mine did), and you can replace your plates, bowls, glasses and cups with glass versions. This is especially important for young children, who are overexposed to plastic sippy cups, teething rings, straws, plates and spoons. Back in the old days, children learned to drink from glass glasses, and I think they're capable of doing the same today.

Unfortunately, all of that pricey non-stick cookware and bakeware you have is bad for your and your child's health because the non-stick coating is an endocrine disruptor. You'll want to replace them with an old-fashioned cast iron skillet (grandma was right!), glass or non-toxic enamel ware.

Check for Mold

Mold in the house can create health problems such as asthma, headaches, nosebleeds and fibromyalgia, and it can exacerbate sensory and gut issues. I've known far too many parents of autistic and SPD children who discovered they had mold in their houses, and the mold was usually hidden in the walls near plumbing that leaked or near poorly constructed weather-proofing. *My House Is Killing Me! The Home Guide for Families with Allergies and Asthma* by Jeffrey C. May and www.survivingmold.com are two great starting points if you suspect your family may have a mold problem in the house. Ritchie Shoemaker of Surviving Mold estimates that 50% of American households have a mold problem.

Eat Organic Food

Food that's not organic is loaded with pesticides, and pesticides cause neurodevelopmental damage. In addition, the Quality Low Input Food Project discovered that organic food contains up to 40% more antioxidants. So if your child is eating non-organic food, he or she is eating more toxins and less antioxidants AND will need to detoxify from the additional toxins.

Organic food by law isn't allowed to contain artificial colors, preservatives or flavors, many of which have been shown to cause neurological and behavioral problems. That doesn't mean that all organic is 100% safe; some synthetic pesticides are still allowed to be used in the production of organic food.[4]

You'll want your child to eat fresh-as-possible organic fruits and vegetables and pasture-raised chickens, eggs, beef and lamb. These types of food not only typically don't contain toxins, but they also have the highest levels of nutrients. If you eat fish, be sure it's either wild-caught, cold-water fish or small fish like sardines that haven't bioaccumulated toxins the way big fish do. At this point, with the Fukushima nuclear plant continually leaking radiation into the Pacific Ocean,[5] I avoid any kind of Pacific fish, including salmon.

Green Your Yard

A great way to reduce your child's exposure to toxins is to stop using pesticides in your yard and house. You won't have a perfect lawn or garden anymore, but your child's health is more important, and it's better for the environment, which ultimately affects all of us. Even if your pesticide company representative tells you that their pesticides are safe, remember that they have a vested interest in selling you their products. There are plenty of safe alternatives, like using cinnamon to deter ants. Also, be sure to have all family members remove their shoes upon entering the house to avoid tracking toxins into the house.

Detoxifying the Body

Now that you've learned about removing toxicity sources from your home and life, it's time to learn how to remove the toxins from your child's body. It is essential that your child is

---

4. U.S. Government Printing Office. Electronic Code of Federal Regulations, Title 7, Subtitle B, Chapter I, Subchapter M, Part 205, Subpart G, The National List of Allowed and Prohibited Substances.
5. http://www.globalresearch.ca/28-signs-that-the-west-coast-is-being-absolutely-fried-with-nuclear-radiation-from-fukushima/5355280 Accessed August 28, 2014.

not chronically constipated or has chronic diarrhea, as the gut is one of the major pathways of elimination. Implementing a gut-healing diet, as discussed earlier, is a great way to clear the gut of dysbiosis that would impair detoxification.

Antioxidants

Toxins such as heavy metals use up a LOT of antioxidants, so you'll want your child to eat as many brightly colored fruits and vegetables because the fresher, less cooked and brighter (natural color, please!) they are, the more antioxidants they have. "Eating the rainbow" of naturally colorful food provides your child with high levels of naturally occurring antioxidants and other phytonutrients.

In addition, you'll want your child to eat a wide variety of herbs and spices such as oregano, rosemary, thyme, turmeric, garlic, basil and cloves because not only do they taste good, but many of them are also antimicrobial as well as being high in antioxidants. Turmeric specifically is one of the most well-studied spices because of its high antioxidant levels.[6]

Food is the best source of antioxidants, but many times, our child's body needs more than he or she can eat, so supplementation can help. Vitamin C in particular helps recycle glutathione, the body's master antioxidant, and it is a water-soluble vitamin, so there is less concern with toxicity because the excess comes out in urine. Royal camu is an excellent natural source of vitamin C.

Vitamin A and vitamin E are also antioxidants, but because they are fat-soluble, your child should only take them in supplement form under the care of a doctor. Instead, opt for nutrient-dense eggs, animal organs, meat and seafood. Dr. Weston A. Price believed that "neither protein, minerals nor

---

6. Ji, Sayer. 600 Reasons Turmeric May Be The World's Most Important Herb, http://www.greenmedinfo.com/blog/600-reasons-turmeric-may-be-worlds-most-important-herb. Accessed August 28, 2014.

water-soluble vitamins can be utilized by the body without vitamin A from animal sources."[7]

Glutathione

Glutathione is the body's super antioxidant, and it helps get rid of heavy metals, especially mercury. The problem with mercury poisoning, though, which is common in many children with Sensory Processing Disorder, is that mercury inhibits the production of glutathione, thereby stopping the body's elimination mechanism, so mercury accumulates in the body.

There is controversy over whether consuming glutathione as a supplement is helpful, and I've heard from other practitioners that the cream is more effective than an oral supplement. Instead of taking glutathione as a supplement, your child can eat the foods containing its amino-acid precursors like glycine, glutamic acid and cysteine. Vegetable sources don't have a lot of these amino acids, but the best vegetable sources are artichokes, asparagus, onions, garlic, spinach, cruciferous vegetables, avocados and spinach.

Animal sources are much better sources of these precursors. Raw, grass-fed milk and raw, organic or pasture-raised eggs are the best sources of cysteine, a glutathione precursor. Raw milk hasn't been pasteurized, so heat hasn't denatured the whey in it. Raw milk is hard to find because different states have different laws on the sale and distribution of it, but you can check out www.realmilk.com to see where you can buy it locally. It is fairly easy to buy raw milk cheeses; you just have to check out the label. I know Whole Foods has quite a few of them; they're usually European. The Weston A. Price Foundation is a non-profit whose goal is to provide information about traditional foods, including raw milk, and why they are better for your health.

---

7. Fallon, Sally and Enig, Mary. "Vitamin Primer". The Weston A. Price Foundation. http://www.westonaprice.org/health-topics/abcs-of-nutrition/vitamin-primer/. Accessed August 24, 2014.

Cultured raw milk products like kefir, yogurt, and sour cream (without sugar, please!) are an even better source of glutathione, as they also provide immune-boosting probiotics. I don't recommend store-bought versions of these because they're pasteurized, because they're not fermented for long enough, because they're typically made with low-fat or no-fat milk and because they also typically contain unwanted and sometimes harmful fillers. I recommend that if your child can tolerate fermented dairy products that you make them yogurt or kefir yourself from raw milk using appropriate starter cultures.

Children who drink raw milk are less likely to develop asthma and allergies than those who stick to the safer pasteurized version.[8] The protective effect was linked to whey proteins in the milk that may be destroyed by pasteurization.

Ann Louise Gittleman says that both gluten (the protein found in wheat, barley, rye, and spelt) and casein (the protein found in dairy products) interfere with cysteine uptake, and therefore interfere with glutathione production. She also says that's why the two allergies seem to go together: if you're allergic to one, you're probably allergic, intolerant or sensitive to the other. However, she does say that raw dairy is outstanding, unless one has a true dairy allergy, which, in her experience is usually due to an underlying parasitical infection.

Sulfur

Sulfur-containing foods are another heavy-hitting source of detoxification, but a high-grain diet and/or a high-processed-food diet are likely to be deficient in sulfur, as processing removes the sulfur.

Sulfur is found in eggs, animal meats, seafood, onions, garlic, asparagus, coconut oil, olive oil, wheat germ and legumes; again, pasture-raised meats and eggs will have the

---

8. Loss, Georg, et al, The protective effect of farm milk consumption on childhood asthma and atopy: The GABRIELA study, *J Allergy Clin Immunol.* 2011 Oct;128(4):766-773.e4

highest amounts of nutrients, including sulfur. Cruciferous vegetables are famous for their sulfur content: broccoli, cauliflower, kale, cabbage, bok choy, cabbage, rutabaga, turnips, kohlrabi, mustards and Brussel sprouts. As an added bonus, cruciferous veggies also contain significant amounts of vitamin C, selenium, indole-3-carbinol (which blocks the growth of cancer cells) and sulforaphane, which not only inhibits cancer cell growth but also is a precursor to glutathione, thereby boosting its production. Broccoli sprouts contain the highest levels of sulforaphane.

Taking a bath in magnesium sulfate (Epsom salts) is another excellent way to get sulfur into your child's body.

Stephanie Seneff is a senior scientist at MIT who studies the health effects of sulfur, among other things. She believes that healthy cholesterol and sulfur levels are highly dependent on vitamin D levels, which is made by exposing your skin to sunshine, so be sure to have your child's vitamin D levels checked.

Herbs

Many herbs are known for their ability to detoxify or protect the body from toxins.

- **Cilantro** removes mercury, aluminum, lead and tin.
- **Turmeric** both detoxifies and also provides an antioxidant effect against mercury.
- **Holy basil** protects against toxicity from mercury.
- **Ginkgo biloba's** antioxidant properties protect against mercury-caused tissue damage.
- **Milk thistle (silymarin)** is full of antioxidants, and it repairs and detoxifies the liver.
- **Dandelion root** is also known for its ability to detoxify the liver.

Probiotics

Probiotics not only protect the liver by preventing intestinal damage, they can also trap and neutralize heavy metals. Some specific strains can reduce organic mercury into a less toxic form.

Supplements

I strongly urge you to have your child see a naturopath or functional-medicine doctor before taking any chelating supplements because if your child binds up (chelates) the heavy metals but doesn't have the means to excrete them, there's just going to be a whole mess of problems. Translation: just because the garbage is getting bagged doesn't mean there's a garbage man around to haul it away, so the garbage is just going to pile up and create a big stinking mess.

In addition, heavy-duty chelating agents are extremely hard on the body, as they not only pull out heavy metals, but they also bind to essential minerals. Chelating can make your child very tired, so if your practitioner performs chelation for your child, make sure he or she is taking extra minerals such as magnesium, selenium, zinc and iodine. Bone broths, vegetables and animal organs are excellent sources of minerals, and organic foods have been shown to have more minerals and nutrients than their pesticide-laden counterparts.

This list is by no means an exhaustive list of detoxification supplements.

- **EDTA** is a heavy-duty chelator that is primarily used to remove lead, mercury, aluminum, and cadmium.
- **DMPS** is another heavy-duty supplement that chelates zinc, copper, arsenic, mercury, cadmium, silver, lead and tin.
- **DMSA** is another heavy-duty chelator, mainly used for lead and mercury elimination.
- **Vitamin C** (and other antioxidants) help gluthathione do

its job better by taking care of most free radicals, thereby saving glutathione for the heavy-metal cleanup.

- **Iodine** keeps the thyroid working properly. If it's not, the liver isn't detoxifying well.
- **Selenium** protects against liver and kidney damage from heavy metals and is necessary for proper thyroid function.
- **Chlorella** and **spirulina** are two different algaes with antioxidants that help remove cadmium and mercury. In addition, they are highly alkalizing.
- **Quercetin**, found in apples, cruciferous vegetables, red onions, capers and numerous other foods, has a protective effect against damage from methylmercury.
- **DHA** may act as a neuroprotective agent against methylmercury's neurotoxicity. Eating saturated fat helps with the absorption of DHA.
- **Astaxanthin** protects against lipid peroxidation from mercury poisoning.
- **L-arginine** is an amino acid that has been shown to reduce mercury accumulation in the thymus.
- **N-acetyl cysteine** is both a precursor to glutathione and an effective heavy-metal chelator.
- **Alpha lipoic acid** and its cousin **R-lipoic acid** (which Dr. Sherry Rogers says is the more active form) have the ability to regenerate glutathione. It also is a sulfur compound that can chelate heavy metals.
- **MSM**, short for methylsulfonylmethane, is an organic form of sulfur and a potent antioxidant.
- **MCP** is modified citrus pectin, which is taken from the pith of citrus fruits. Research studies showed that MCP is an effective and gentle heavy-metal chelator[9, 10].
- **Clays such as bentonite and zeolite** have molecules that are negatively charged, which attracts them to the positive charges of heavy metals.

---

9. Zhao, ZY, et al, The role of modified citrus pectin as an effective chelator of lead in children hospitalized with toxic lead levels, *Altern Ther Health* Med. 2008 Jul-Aug;14(4):34-8.
10. Eliaz, I, The effect of modified citrus pectin on urinary excretion of toxic elements, *Phytother Res.* 2006 Oct;20(10):859-64.

Juicing

Juicing fruits and vegetables is an effective and immediate way to get phytonutrients and antioxidants into your child for detoxification. Juicing can be an easy way for your child to get involved in choosing what he or she eats; carrots and apples are a great place to start for children. My children love to help me juice. I chop up the fruits and vegetables to be juiced into small pieces, and they have fun putting the food into the chute and watching it come out.

Alkalinization

By alkalizing your child's body, you'll make it easier to flush out toxins. An acidic body condition easily leads to diseases and disorders, and most of us are in a constantly acidic state due to stresses from environmental toxins, emotional stress, EMFs and the food we eat or don't eat. Be sure to check the pH of your child's saliva with a pH test strip, as the optimal pH for maximum detoxification is 7.0 to 7.4.

There are many ways to alkalize:

- Minerals, which come from:
    - Vegetables
    - Unrefined salt: sea salt, Himalayan salt or Real Salt
    - Bone broths
    - Liver and other animal organs
    - Supplements
- Raw apple cider vinegar
- Lemon juice
- Eating less acidic foods such as sugar, meat and cheese
- Baking soda
- Practice de-stressing techniques such as:
    - Listening to classical music
    - Meditating
    - Being in nature

- Praying
- Yoga

Juicing, as discussed above, is a great way to get in more phytonutrients and antioxidants, but it's also a great way for your child to alkalize. Putting a little fresh lemon juice in their drinking water between meals can help, too. Having your child bathe in raw apple cider vinegar, Epsom salts, Dead Sea salts and/or baking soda can help as well, although I don't recommend putting vinegar and baking soda into the tub at the same time!

Clay Baths

Having your child take a clay bath is an easy and gentle way to detoxify without asking them to ingest a multitude of supplements. LL's Magnetic Clay offers a variety of clay bath kits to help your child detoxify from things such as radiation, arsenic, aluminum, formaldehyde, mercury, lead and copper.

Exercise

A good, sweaty spell of running around and playing is one of the best ways for your SPD child to detoxify. Young children under the age of eight lack the ability to sweat a whole lot, however.

Homeopathy

Homeopathy is a very safe form of healing based on the principle of like cures like, or "the hair of the dog that bit you is the cure for what ails you." Homeopathic remedies contain infinitesimally small amounts of a substance that give the body just enough information to tell it how to heal. At such a small amount, the remedy is really more of an energetic imprint.

I discovered homeopathy for myself after getting a very bad body-covering poison ivy rash. At that time, I was seeing a typical Western-medicine doctor, and she gave me a six-pack of steroids, which made the rash go away until I stopped taking them; then the rash came back with a vengeance. I didn't want to take more steroids, so I did my research and discovered homeopathic poison ivy, *Rhus toxiconderon*, at Whole Foods. It made the rash go away without the nasty side effects that steroids have. After that, I was hooked.

Homeopathy can be used to correct imbalances as well as to detoxify. Homeopathic heavy-metal detox solutions, such as HVS Labs' Detoxosode, are effective and gentle chelators. If you take your child to a homeopath, he or she can develop a custom solution for your child's issues. For an in-depth discussion of how homeopathy can be used for a neurodevelopmental disorder, in this case ADHD, I recommend Stephen Cowan, MD's book, *Fire Child, Water Child: How Understanding the Five Types of ADHD Can Help You Improve Your Child's Self-Esteem & Attention.*

Homeopathy can also be used for the relief of chronic and acute health problems. I prefer to use homeopathic remedies instead of pharmaceuticals because pharmaceuticals always have side effects. Homeopathy is very safe and can be used to shift the overall health of your family for the better. I use homeopathic remedies for things like colds, coughs, runny noses and pain, and a great resource for learning more about this is *Your Natural Medicine Cabinet, A Practical Guide to Drug-Free Remedies for Common Ailments* by Burke Lennihan, RN, CCH.

CEASE Therapy

A special type of homeopathy directed at detoxifying children from vaccines, environmental toxins and other causes of neurodevelopmental damage is CEASE therapy, which stands for Complete Elimination of Autism Spectrum Expression. Your SPD child may or may not be on the autism spectrum, but don't worry about the labels because the perfect storm of causes is the same. This specialized therapy was developed by Tinus Smits, MD, and you can find out more about it at www.cease-therapy.com and from his book, *Autism, Beyond Despair: CEASE Therapy, Homeopathy Has the Answers.*

Vibrational Remedies

Vibrational remedies are similar to homeopathy in that they balance out an energetic imbalance, many of which are caused by miasms, which are energetic taints on DNA that can get passed down through generations. In addition, many of these imbalances can be caused by environmental toxins such as vaccines, pesticides and radiation, and vibrational remedies can clear and detoxify your child safely and easily.

Michelle Giliberto is a vibrational therapy practitioner of Healers Who Share, and she is also one of the co-founders of Epidemic Answers, the non-profit for which I work. Michelle recovered her son from autism and her daughter from Lyme disease with a combination of dietary changes, biomedical treatment and vibrational remedies. You can read her children's recovery story here: www.epidemicanswers.org /recovery/lyme-autism-recovery/

Things to Remember

Before you do any major detoxification, you need to make sure your child's channels of elimination (pee, poop, sweat and lungs) are open. I highly recommend working with a naturopath for this because they are far more knowledgeable about this than any other type of doctor I've seen. You don't want all those heavy metals and other toxins recirculating in your child's body after you've tried to remove them.

The two best books that I've read (so far) about how to detoxify from heavy metals and other toxins, especially plasticizers, BPA and pesticides, are Sherry Rogers, MD's' *Detoxify or Die* and Mark Hyman MD's/Mark Liponis MD's *Ultraprevention: The 6-Week Plan That Will Make You Healthy for*

Life. Dr. Rogers has a great newsletter called "Total Wellness" in which she explains why current medical dogma will harm you, and Dr. Hyman's website www.drhyman.com is a great online resource for understanding the role of toxins and how diet can help you detoxify.

ADDRESSING RESIDUAL ISSUES

You may find that your child has residual health issues even after going through all of the steps to recover him or her from his symptoms. That's normal! There are so many layers to this onion, and everyone is different. After recovering my sons from Sensory Processing Disorder, I discovered my older son had subclinical cystic fibrosis, which was the real reason for his failure to thrive, as well as his asthma. Mitochondrial dysfunction was responsible for my younger's son's failure to thrive. Because it is such a key, common issue to just about any disease or disorder, I'm going to explore it here in more detail.

Looking at Mitochondrial Dysfunction

The best way to think of mitochondrial dysfunction is like thinking about economics: supply and demand. People with mitochondrial dysfunctions can't supply enough energy to meet their bodies' demands. Seemingly typical things to most people can cause an energy drain in these people. Illness and stress of any kind (even if you think it's no big deal) can place a huge energy drain on a body that has trouble supplying it, and the body "crashes" with symptoms like fatigue, pain, nausea and GI system shutdown.

Here are some common causes of energy drains:

- Stress
- Being in a noisy, crowded environment
- Emotional stress
- Hypoglycemia
- Heat and humidity
- Too-cold temperatures
- Hormonal fluctuations
- Illness
- Too much physical activity
- Demands of school (a lot of fine-motor activity, writing)

At this point, you're probably scratching your head, thinking "Mitochondria… I vaguely remember something about that from high school biology class." Mitochondria are the powerhouses of the cells. They make energy from our food, and if they are gunked up or damaged, they don't work properly, and you feel tired, shaky or sick.

Dr. Doug Wallace,[1] director of the Center of Mitochondrial and Epigenomic Medicine at the Children's Hospital of Philadelphia, says that energy is life and that all disease has its roots in mitochondrial dysfunction, as he wrote in this article for the journal *Genetics*: "Mitochondria as Chi."[2]

The College of American Pathologists says that, "Mitochondrial dysfunctions are the Willy Lomans of disease – difficult to fathom, easy to overlook, dropping hints that don't quite add up to a full portrait." Their article, "Untangling the Knot of Mitochondrial Dysfunction,"[3] gives a great overview

---

1. http://www.ninds.nih.gov/recovery/arra-stories/wallace_mitos_autism.htm. Accessed August, 26, 2014.
2. Wallace, Douglas. Mitochondria as Chi. *Genetics*, June 2008 vol. 179 no. 2 727-735
3. http://www.captodayonline.com/cap_today_september_091911.html.

of what mitochondrial disease is and why it's so difficult to pin down.

Symptoms of Mitochondrial Dysfunction

Mitochondrial dysfunction can cause a host of symptoms. Having symptoms across three or more organ systems is suggestive of mitochondrial dysfunction:

- Seizures
- Lack of energy, low stamina
- Failure to thrive
- Muscle pain, spasms and cramping
- Hypotonia
- Memory and concentration issues
- Heat intolerance
- Developmental delays
- Lack of coordination
- Constipation
- Acid reflux
- Slow motility, gastroparesis
- Nausea
- Migraines/headaches
- Dizziness
- Malabsorption
- Immunodeficiency
- Sleep issues and dysfunctions
- Difficulty recovering from fever, illness or anesthesia
- Pancreatic insufficiency

Mitochondrial dysfunction causes an overabundance of metabolic by-products, high levels of which are red flags for mitochondrial dysfunction: lactic acid, pyruvic acid, alinine and lysine. Checking the levels of carnitine, lactic acid, pyruvic acid, alinine and lysine are easy preliminary screening tests that

---

Accessed August 26, 2014.

can be done from a standard blood-test lab like Quest Diagnostics.

Carnitine is a conditionally essential amino acid that's used to transport fatty acids into the cell to be used as fuel for energy production. It comes from the Latin word "carne," which means flesh, and, indeed, beef and pork are excellent sources of it. Not having enough carnitine means there aren't enough conveyor belts for fuel into the cells.

An over-accumulation of lactic acid, as many athletes know, causes muscle cramps and spasms. Lactic acid will increase significantly when a person with mitochondrial dysfunction is ill.

These preliminary tests cannot confirm a diagnosis. They are only screening tests for the next level of tests, such as muscle biopsy and genetic screening, that can be used to make a diagnosis, which can be tricky and elusive. Muscle biopsy is painful, expensive ($15,000), invasive and requires anesthesia, which is a significant concern in kids with mitochondrial dysfunction, and genetic testing is expensive ($5,000).

In maternally inherited mitochondrial disease, mothers are also affected, so if you discover your child has some form of mitochondrial dysfunction, you'll want to get yourself screened, too.

Causes of Mitochondrial Dysfunction

Mitochondrial dysfunction can come from genetic inheritance or exposure to environmental toxins, medications or other triggers. If it's inherited, it can come from mom (which is known as maternal inheritance) or it can be autosomal recessive and be inherited from both mom and dad.

Sherry Rogers, MD believes that mitochondrial damage comes mostly from environmental toxins such as plasticizers, pesticides[4] and heavy metals. She states that when

4. de la Asunción JG, et al, AZT induces oxidative damage to cardiac mitochondria: protective effect of vitamins C and E, *Life Sci.* 2004 Nov 19;76(1):47-56.

mitochondria develop leaky membranes, this is "the basis for all disease" because "the very essence of life (energy from food) is created in the mitochondria."[5]

Andrew Cutler, PhD, also believes that heavy metals, specifically mercury, cause mitochondrial damage. Dental amalgams, or "silver" fillings that are actually 50% mercury, are the largest source of mercury in our bodies today. You can find out more about his heavy metal chelation protocol at his website www.noamalgam.com and in his book, *Amalgam Illness: Diagnosis and Treatment: A Book on How to Cure Mercury Poisoning.*

Environmental toxins are passed from the mother to the fetus. The Environmental Working Group published a landmark report back in 2005 titled, "Body Burden – The Pollution in Newborns." This report showed that a total of 287, and an average of over 200, toxins were found in the cord blood of newborns, meaning that they could only come from the mother.

Toxins bio-accumulate over time and across generations. Every generation along the way accumulates its own set of toxins, and the toxic burden is compounded. We've reached the point where the toxic burden is so high that our babies are being born "pre-polluted," as the Body Burden report says.

However, just so you know, it is not widely accepted by the western medicine mitochondrial community that heavy metals cause or are part of mitochondrial dysfunction, but there is increasing consensus that mitochondrial disease can be "triggered" by chemicals or physiological stress and can be made worse by alcohol consumption (especially binge drinking), cigarettes and MSG. The meta-study, "Mitochondrial Regulation of Epigenetics and Its Role in Human Diseases,"[6] looks at a number of studies that look into how toxins can damage mitochondrial DNA or even nuclear

---

5. Stavrovskaya IG, The powerhouse takes control of the cell: is the mitochondrial permeability transition a viable therapeutic target against neuronal dysfunction and death?, *Free Radic Biol Med.* 2005 Mar 15;38(6):687-97.

6. Minocherhomji S, Mitochondrial regulation of epigenetics and its role in human diseases, *Epigenetics.* 2012 Apr;7(4):326-34

DNA, leading them to trigger diseases for which a person may be predisposed.

Classically trained geneticists believe that mitochondrial disease is inherited maternally (there are 13 known dysfunctions: POLG, LHON, MELAS, etc.) or is autosomal recessive (one from the mother and one from the father). Historically, these were thought to be rare and neurodegenerative, so this is the basic thinking of MOST mainstream, western medicine geneticists: that mitochondrial disease is rare and that you cannot stabilize these people. But because of what we have learned from others (Dr. Doug Wallace, Dr. Sherry Rogers, Dr. Andrew Cutler, Dr. Richard Boles and more), this thinking may soon change. They believe that mitochondrial dysfunction is not "rare." They believe it's really quite common because it has its roots in MANY illnesses today.

Risk Factors for Mitochondrial Dysfunction?

Mitochondrial dysfunction is common in children with:

- Developmental delays
- Autism
- PDD-NOS
- Sensory Processing Disorder

Given the overlap of conditions, symptoms and people that most likely have mitochondrial dysfunction and given that mitochondrial dysfunction can be caused by environmental toxicity, it's possible that methylation defects are also to blame. Methylation defects are common in people with autism, ADHD, allergies, asthma, SPD, autoimmune diseases and more. A methylation defect means that you're not able to detoxify properly, and, in fact, toxins typically pile up, leading to a whole host of symptoms, conditions and diseases similar to what's seen in people with mitochondrial dysfunction.

Solutions for Mitochondrial Dysfunction

People with mitochondrial disease usually take what's known as the "mito cocktail." It's a mix of vitamins, minerals and other nutrients that are given at therapeutic doses to boost a person's energy level. A first line of supplementation usually contains CoQ10, carnitine and creatine, riboflavin (vitamin B_2) as well as other B vitamins, and an antioxidant component of vitamins C and E.

Often, OTC carnitine is initially recommended, but oftentimes, it's not bioavailable enough or potent enough to make a difference. If that doesn't make a difference, a prescription version of it called Carnitor is given; the generic is called levocarnitine. Children with a history of seizures shouldn't take carnitine, as it can increase the risk of seizures.[7]

Some MDs also use thiamine (vitamin B_1), alpha lipoic acid, folinic acid and selenium. Go to www.umdf.org to see what tier one and tier two supplements are frequently used to treat mitochondrial disorders but be aware that each person's cocktail tends to vary based on symptoms, labs and supervising physician.

The only proven treatment for people with mitochondrial dysfunction at this time is exercise, so it's important to get kids that have some form of it moving and active, which is tough when the child is fatigued.

Further Resources

There are some great resources out there for those wanting to know more about mitochondrial dysfunction. The first is www.mitoaction.org, which is the website for a non-profit organization whose goals are to support, educate and advocate for those with mitochondrial disease. They "are a

7. http://umm.edu/health/medical/altmed/supplement/carnitine-lcarnitine. Accessed September 25, 2014.

committee of parents, patients and clinicians from top Boston hospitals who care about improving the daily quality of life for all people affected by mitochondrial disease."

There are also quarterly free tele-conferences for parents looking for information on the connection between mitochondrial disease and autism. This is an opportunity for families to connect with people knowledgeable about mitochondrial disease. You can find this link at www.mitoaction.org/autism.

The Executive Director of MitoAction, Cristy Balcells, wrote an excellent book called *Living Well with Mitochondrial Disease: A Handbook for Patients, Parents, and Families.* It's the one book you need if you want to learn about mitochondrial disease from soup to nuts.

There is a lot of excellent information available on the United Mitochondrial Disease Foundation (UMDF) website at www.umdf.org.

Our Mito Story

Our pediatrician sent us to see Vicki Kobliner, a holistic nutritionist, who's also on the board of Epidemic Answers with me, for Crane Man's (my younger son's) failure to thrive. Given that Crane Man had constant fatigue and stomach pain, poor growth, mild sensory issues and developmental delays, Vicki suggested having preliminary tests for mitochondrial dysfunction done.

Crane Man's developmental delay was a symptom of brain dysfunction; his GI problems and former acid reflux were symptoms of muscular dysfunction; his possible hypoglycemia was a symptom of liver dysfunction; and his failure to thrive, fatigue and former unexplained vomiting were symptoms of system dysfunction.

Crane Man's total carnitine level was at 12umol/L; the lowest normal level is 32. Free carnitine was 10; the lowest normal level is 25. His lactic acid level was 8, which was in the normal range of 4-16mg/dL, so there was no problem there with him. However, Crane Man's pyruvic acid level was high at

1.63; the high normal range is 1.50mg/dL, so that is a definite red flag.

There was a miscommunication with the lab, and the wrong test was ordered for his alinine and lysine levels. Given that he had at least 15 vials taken for his regular blood panels and these newer tests, I decided to forego having him tested for these other amino acids at this time, especially since his carnitine and pyruvic acid levels suggest he may have mitochondrial dysfunction.

Imagine my shock when these preliminary tests suggested Crane Man has mitochondrial dysfunction. Let me be clear here and say that I am not talking about the classical, rare, neurodegenerative disease, but rather what's called a "functional mitochondrial disorder," as Dr. Richard Boles wrote about.[8]

It makes sense that Crane Man has an energy imbalance because his weight-percentile decline coincided perfectly with his going to preschool. In other words, he stopped gaining weight at his typical rate once he started preschool even though he was eating about the same amount of food. I'm wondering if just the emotional stress of being separated from me and being in a new environment were more stress on him than he could handle. Poor baby!

Once I found out that Crane Man likely had mitochondrial dysfunction, I immediately requested tests for my older son, who has borne the brunt of the health problems between the two of them, such as more-severe SPD, acid reflux, asthma, allergies, eczema, developmental delays, fatigue and hypotonia. When he was little, he was so limp that he was like a limp Raggedy Andy doll. My older son's tests also indicate he may have mitochondrial dysfunction, as his carnitine level is below the normal range at 20 and his lactic acid level is above the range at 17. No wonder he often wakes up with muscle cramps.

---

8. http://www.mitoaction.org/blog/dr-richard-boles-functional-mitochondrial-disorders. Accessed August 26, 2014.

EMPOWERING YOURSELF

My goal in writing this book is to teach you how to take back the power that we've given over to others so that you can recover the health of your child.

Becoming Your Child's Advocate

No one else knows your child as well as you do, and no one else has his or her best interests at heart as much as you do. It's time to do your own research. You have to stand up for your child, even if it means leaving a pediatric practice or educating your child's doctors about what's going on with your child.

SPD is not a psychiatric condition; it's a whole-body condition that affects the way the brain functions. Most pediatricians and other doctors are not aware of this; it's not in their education, so it's up to you to educate yourself and them. You can give them a copy of this book to help educate them. Knowledge is power. And once you learn this, you can't "unknow" it.

Doing Your Own Research

I'm fortunate because I used to be an equity research analyst on Wall Street and a marketing analyst for an oil-services firm before that, so I know how to research issues. My mom was an information analyst for the Department of Energy at Oak Ridge National Lab, where the first atomic bomb was made, so I must have picked the ability up from her.

I urge you to be very selective in where you get your health news. If it's from the mainstream media like TV news, newspapers and magazines, you have to remember that nothing is going to be said or written that is too controversial.

They know who butters their bread, and a significant chunk of that butter comes from ads from pharmaceutical companies and even Big Ag companies, whose interest is not in keeping you healthy; it's in making money for themselves from you buying their products.

I find my best sources to be books and newsletters because they are well researched and because you can independently review the research that is referenced. I particularly like Sherry Rogers, MD's' "Total Wellness" newsletter as she references her articles to the nth degree.

When I read a book, I also look at the list of scientific papers and books that are listed in the resource section in the book, which gives me a whole other set of publications from where I can learn more.

Establishing a Game Plan

It's an overwhelming task for many parents to even think of recovering their child from Sensory Processing Disorder. My advice is to take it one step at a time. If you have a setback, shake it off and keep going. No one is 100% perfect 100% of the time. This is not about perfection; it's about consistency.

If you implement the changes I've told you about, you can get a real leg up on recovering your child. Making dietary changes can be a chore, but it's also empowering to know that you can make such a big difference in your child's life. Getting proper nutrition into your child is key to improving outcomes for any other therapies you try. As far as I know, no child has recovered fully without making dietary changes. Don't kill yourself thinking that is how your child will have to eat for the rest of their lives. You're looking at a two-to-three year hump after which you can let your guard down a little. The more you put into this, the more you'll get out of it!

Finding a Practitioner

Once you've started to make the changes I recommend, then you'll need help finding a skilled practitioner. I recommend working with a naturopath, integrative or functional-medicine doctor first, although these kinds can be few and far between. At Epidemic Answers, we've put together a database of providers to help you with your search. Right now, the list is small and doesn't include providers in every state, but it's growing. You can find it at www.epidemicanswers.org. Remember, just because a provider lists "autism" or "ADHD" as a specialty, don't think they can't help your child because they can.

Reaching Out to Others

Finding likeminded parents on their recovery journey is key to helping you maintain your momentum. When you start implementing the changes I've recommended, it's going to be difficult for you and your family socially because you'll be scrutinizing the food at birthday parties and get-togethers. It helps to find someone that is going through what you're going through or has already been there. Facebook groups are a great way to meet people from all over the world to share your experiences with. Local meetups of Holistic Moms' Network are another option.

Learning More

Hopefully, once you start this journey, your quest for learning more will become insatiable! I know it did for me. I've listed tons of resources – books, movies, DVDs, websites and newsletters – in the back of the book for you, but I want to point out a few that are good starting points:

- Epidemic Answers: www.epidemicanswers.org
- Talk About Curing Autism: www.tacanow.org
- The Thinking Moms' Revolution: www.thinkingmomsrevolution.com
- Fearless Parent: www.fearlesparent.org
- Developmental Delay Resources: www.devdelay.org

Using the Oxygen Mask

If you're a mom reading this book and working on recovering your child, it's likely that you have your own set of health problems, many of which are similar to your child's issues. Most moms of special needs kids have PTSD: permanent traumatic stress disorder. It doesn't stop! You've got to learn to put the oxygen mask on yourself first and take care of yourself so you can help your child better. As a health coach, I work with the whole family to help recover a child. I especially emphasize the overlap between moms and their kids, and I don't charge extra for it because moms are usually the ones bearing the brunt of this. They're usually the ones schlepping their children to therapists and doctors, doing the grocery shopping and cooking the food. Mom may as well get some benefit!

Demonstrating Evidence of Hope

I want to let you know what the Canary Kids Project means to me: hope. By making this film in which we will document the potential recovery of 14 children from autism, ADHD, asthma, atopic dermatitis, mood disorders, juvenile rheumatoid arthritis and type 2 diabetes, I believe people will come to know what I do: that recovery is possible. If you know that recovery is possible, then you have hope.

In this film, we'll be rigorously documenting the therapies, lab work, diets, healing modalities and biomedical approaches that are used in each child's healing protocol.

I wish something like this had been around when my boys were younger. Back then, it was enough for me to figure out finally that they had Sensory Processing Disorder, which I call "autism light" or "almost autism."

It took loads of research on my end to understand that their developmental delays, hypotonia, asthma, allergies, eczema, failure to thrive, projectile vomiting and acid reflux were all related.

It took even more researching and networking to discover that recovery from autism is possible. If kids can be recovered from autism, and Sensory Processing Disorder is like a subset of autism, then my boys could be recovered from SPD.

I discovered a hidden world of what's called the "biomedical" approach to healing, which is what functional medicine is: Getting to the root cause of a symptom, illness or disorder.

The problem was, and is, that most doctors just don't know about this type of approach. Thankfully, functional-medicine doctors like Dr. Mark Hyman, Dr. Susan Blum and Dr. Frank Lipman are showing us that food is medicine and that toxicity, gut dysbiosis, hormonal imbalances and nutritional deficiencies are the ultimate causes of just about any kind of chronic disease or disorder.

JUMPING IN

You may be overwhelmed at the thought of implementing all of these changes. That's where I come in. I'll be the guide on your side to help you make all of these diet and lifestyle tweaks. All of these little changes can and do make a big difference.

I'd love to help you recover your child. I can point you in the right direction when you get stuck, be your sounding board when you need someone to listen to you so you don't feel crazy about what you're doing, be a cheerleader for you and help you make all of these changes. It's a lot to take on, but you can do it!

If you'd like to speak with me about how I can help you, you can go to my website and pick a time and date that work for your consultation by going to:
www.mariarickerthong.com/consultation

INVITING ME TO SPEAK

I love to speak about the epidemic of children's chronic illnesses and about recovery. If your group or organization would like to have me speak at your next event, please let me know by going to my website and filling out my "Contact Me" form at: www.mariarickerthong.com/contact-me

RECIPES

Amaranth Porridge

Serves:	4
Cook time:	30 minutes
Allergy:	tree nuts
Special diets:	dairy-free, diabetic, egg-free, gluten-free, vegan, vegetarian
Meal type:	breakfasts, grains
Miscellaneous:	freezable, pre-preparable, serve hot

This easy-to-make amaranth porridge for breakfast uses an often-overlooked gluten-free grain with a nutty flavor.

Ingredients

1 cup amaranth (soaked overnight, rinsed and drained)
2-1/2 cups cold, filtered water
1 cup berries
4 tablespoons raw, local honey
4 tablespoons walnut oil
1 teaspoon ground cinnamon (I prefer Celyon cinnamon)
1 teaspoon sea salt

Directions

Place amaranth and water in a 2 quart pot with a lid. Bring to a boil then reduce heat to low and simmer for between 20 and 30 minutes or until liquid has been absorbed. Stir in remaining ingredients and serve.

Arugula Salad with Fennel and Orange

Serves:	4
Prep time:	15 minutes
Cook time:	5 minutes
Total time:	20 minutes
Special diets:	dairy-free, GAPS/SCD, gluten-free, Paleo
Meal type:	salads
Miscellaneous:	serve cold

To supreme an orange, slice off the peel to remove the pith, then cut into each wedge and pull out just the pulpy part, leaving the skin of the wedge attached to the core.

Ingredients

3 oranges
1 lemon (juiced)
1 tablespoon raw apple cider vinegar
1 tablespoon extra-virgin olive oil
1/2 teaspoon sea salt
1 fennel bulb (thinly sliced)
16 mushrooms (thinly sliced)
1 red onion (thinly sliced)
6oz arugula
3 slices bacon (cooked and crumbled)

Directions

Supreme 2 oranges. Juice the other one and mix with lemon juice, vinegar, olive oil and sea salt. Mix fennel, mushrooms, onion and spinach in a large bowl. Toss with vinaigrette. Put on individual serving plates and top with bacon.

Coconut Chia Pudding

Serves:	2
Prep time:	2 minutes
Special diets:	dairy-free, diabetic, egg-free, GAPS/SCD, gluten-free, Paleo, vegan, vegetarian
Meal type:	desserts, snacks
Miscellaneous:	child-friendly, pre-preparable, serve cold

I use vanilla bean powder for depth of flavor and also so I can skip the alcohol in this super-easy coconut chia pudding recipe. It's Paleo-, GAPS- and SCD-legal.

Ingredients

1 cup full-fat coconut milk
6 tablespoons chia seeds
1/2 teaspoon vanilla bean powder

Directions

Combine all ingredients in a lidded jar. Shake a few times. Refrigerate for at least 30 minutes. Top with your favorite fruit!

Coconut Cream Blonde Macaroons

Serves:	24
Prep time:	5 minutes
Cook time:	25 minutes
Total time:	30 minutes
Special diets:	dairy-free, GAPS/SCD, gluten-free, vegetarian
Meal type:	desserts
Miscellaneous:	child-friendly, pre-preparable, serve cold

Ingredients

1 cup coconut cream (I like "Let's Do... Organic")
2 cups shredded, unsweetened coconut
3/4 cups raw, local honey
1-1/4 teaspoon vanilla extract
1/2 teaspoon almond extract
1/2 teaspoon fine sea salt

Directions

Blend all ingredients in a food processor or blender. Bake for 20-25 minutes in a 300° Fahrenheit oven or dehydrate at 118° Fahrenheit for 24 hours.

Coconut-Cream Scrambled Eggs

Serves:	4
Prep time:	5 minutes
Cook time:	5 minutes
Total time:	10 minutes
Allergy:	egg
Special diets:	dairy-free, diabetic, GAPS/SCD, gluten-free, Paleo, vegetarian
Meal type:	breakfasts
Miscellaneous:	child-friendly, serve hot

Eggs from pastured hens contain more vitamin A, vitamin E, omega-3 fatty acids and beta carotene than factory-farmed eggs.

Ingredients

2 tablespoons creamed coconut (I like "Let's Do… Organic")
1/4 cup filtered water
6 large pasture-raised eggs
2 teaspoons ghee, pastured butter or coconut oil (if you want a dairy-free version, use either ghee or coconut oil)
Sea salt (to taste)

Directions

Chop off 2 tablespoons of creamed coconut from the block of creamed coconut. Put in saucepan with 1/4 c. filtered water. Simmer until creamed coconut has dissolved. Preheat skillet; melt butter. Add creamed coconut to whisked eggs. Whisk together. Pour into skillet and cook until desired consistency.

Coconut-Lemongrass Butternut Squash Soup

Serves:	16
Prep time:	15 minutes
Cook time:	30 minutes
Total time:	45 minutes
Special diets:	dairy-free, diabetic, GAPS/SCD, gluten-free, Paleo, vegan, vegetarian
Meal type:	soups
Miscellaneous:	freezable, pre-preparable, serve hot
Occasion:	casual party

This hearty, creamy soup is fast and easy to make, yet still has a rich flavor without using dairy

Ingredients

2 tablespoons ghee or coconut oil
4 large onions
1 head garlic (peeled and chopped)
8 cups homemade broth
1 large butternut squash (peeled, scooped out and cubed)
2 stalks lemongrass (smashed)
2 teaspoons sea salt
1 box (7 oz.) creamed coconut (I like "Let's Do...Organic")

Directions

In a Dutch oven, melt ghee. Sauté onions for 5 minutes; add in garlic and cook for 1 minute longer. Add in broth, followed by the rest of the ingredients. Cover and cook for 30 minutes or until butternut squash is soft. Cool mixture. Remove lemongrass stalks. Puree' in blender or food processor. Serve immediately.

Creamy Fruit Pudding Without the Cream

Serves:	4
Prep time:	5 minutes
Special diets:	dairy-free, diabetic, GAPS/SCD, gluten-free, Paleo, vegan, vegetarian
Meal type:	desserts, snacks
Miscellaneous:	child-friendly, serve cold

This dessert is loaded with healthy fats and antioxidants. You won't believe it's dairy-free, it's so creamy.

Ingredients

2 ripe avocados
10oz frozen fruit (or 2 cups fresh fruit)
1/4 cup raw, local honey
Pinch sea salt
½ teaspoon powdered vanilla bean

Directions

Scoop out avocado pulp, and put it and the other ingredients into a blender. Process until smooth.

Dairy Free Sweet Potatoes

Serves:	8
Prep time:	10 minutes
Cook time:	1 hour, 50 minutes
Total time:	2 hours
Special diets:	dairy-free, egg-free, gluten-free, Paleo, vegan, vegetarian
Meal type:	other vegetables, side dishes
Miscellaneous:	child-friendly, freezable, pre-preparable serve hot
Occasion:	holidays

I use Hannah yams instead of sweet potatoes in this dairy free sweet potatoes dish because they're creamier and not as sweet as regular sweet potatoes.

Ingredients

4 large sweet potatoes
1/4 cup coconut oil or ghee
2 tablespoons coconut milk
1/2 cup applesauce (preferably homemade)
2 teaspoons fresh ginger (peeled and grated)
1 teaspoon sea salt
2 large apples (peeled, cored and sliced into 1-inch slices)

Directions

Preheat oven to 350° Fahrenheit . Arrange potatoes on a baking sheet or Silpat and bake until tender, 80-90 minutes. Remove from oven and cool. Scoop out insides of potatoes and place in electric mixer bowl. Add 2 tablespoons of ghee and coconut milk, and mix on medium speed with paddle attachment until smooth. Add in applesauce, ginger and salt. Transfer mixture to baking dish and bake for 10 minutes. Cook apples in remaining coconut oil until soft, about 10 minutes. Place apples on top of sweet potato mixture and serve.

Easy Beef Bone Broth

Serves:	16
Prep time:	5 minutes
Cook time:	24 hours
Total time:	24 hours, 5 minutes
Special diets:	Body Ecology Diet, dairy-free, diabetic, egg-free, GAPS/SCD, gluten-free, Paleo
Meal type:	soups
Miscellaneous:	child-friendly, freezable, pre-preparable serve hot

I use homemade broth to cook beans, grains and soups or as a stand-alone. You can reuse beef bones a few times to make more broth; it'll just take a little longer each time. For the subsequent broths, add in a tablespoon or two of Great Lakes gelatin, which is so healing to the lining of the gut.

Ingredients

2lb grass-fed beef marrow and/or joint bones
1 teaspoon ghee or animal fat, melted
1 teaspoon white or apple cider vinegar
1 strip kombu (kelp)

Directions

Rub ghee/fat onto beef bones. Bake at 250° Fahrenheit for one hour; turn, and bake for another hour. Add vinegar, kombu and bones to a large crock pot; fill with filtered water. Cook for at least 24 hours on low.

Easy Chicken Broth

Serves:	16
Prep time:	5 minutes
Cook time:	24 hours
Total time:	24 hours, 5 minutes
Special diets:	Body Ecology Diet, dairy-free, diabetic, egg-free, GAPS/SCD, gluten-free, Paleo
Meal type:	soups
Miscellaneous:	child-friendly, freezable, pre-preparable serve hot

Ingredients

Bones of 1 chicken or 10-12 bones (tubular bones should be chopped in half to allow marrow to come out)
1 large onion (roughly chopped)
1 large carrot (roughly chopped)
1 large celery stalk (roughly chopped)
1 teaspoon ghee, pastured butter, coconut oil or other saturated fat (if you want a dairy-free version, use either ghee or coconut oil)
1 teaspoon white or apple cider vinegar
1 strip kombu (kelp)

Directions

Place all ingredients in a roasting pan; toss to coat. Cook in oven at 350° Fahrenheit degrees for 20 minutes. Remove from oven; turn ingredients over to cook other side. Cook for another 20 minutes. Remove from oven and place all ingredients in a crock pot. Fill to top with filtered water. Let cook for at least 24 hours. If you want to make a bone broth even faster, don't cook the bones in the oven. Don't use the fat, and put all ingredients directly into the crockpot.

Garlicky Greens

Serves:	4
Prep time:	10 minutes
Cook time:	5 minutes
Total time:	15 minutes
Special diets:	Body Ecology Diet, dairy-free, diabetic, egg-free, GAPS/SCD, gluten-free, Paleo, vegan, vegetarian
Meal type:	leafy greens
Miscellaneous:	child-friendly, serve hot

Here's how to cook any kind of leafy green vegetable simply and deliciously!

Ingredients

1 bunch leafy green vegetable
1 head garlic (minced. I like a LOT of garlic! You don't have to use this much if you don't want to.)
1 tablespoon extra virgin olive oil
1/4 teaspoon sea salt

Directions

Remove stem from leaf, chop; set aside. If you have collard greens or kale, you will need to blanch the leaves in a pot of boiling water for a few seconds until they turn a bright green. Once they do, shock them by placing in ice water to stop them from cooking further. Chop to desired thickness. Heat oil in large sauté pan over medium low. Sauté garlic for a minute, then add in chopped stems and cook for a few minutes, until soft. For kale or collard greens, add leaves to garlic and stems. Mix thoroughly and remove from heat. For any other type of green (spinach, chard, mustard greens, turnip greens, carrot greens, beet greens, dandelion greens, etc.), shred and place in pan on top of garlic. Keep turning over until all leaves are wilted. Remove from pan and chop to desired thickness.

Gluten-Free Vanilla Wafers

Serves:	36
Prep time:	10 minutes
Cook time:	10 minutes
Total time:	20 minutes
Allergy:	egg
Special diets:	dairy-free, gluten-free, vegetarian
Meal type:	bready foods, desserts
Miscellaneous:	child-friendly, freezable, pre-preparable, serve cold, serve hot

This is a quick, easy recipe for cookies that your kids will love, and they won't even know they're gluten-free!

Ingredients

1/2 cup ghee, pastured butter or coconut oil (melted; if you want a dairy-free version, use either ghee or coconut oil)
1/3 cup raw, local honey
1/2 teaspoon sea salt
3 large pasture-raised eggs
2 tablespoons vanilla extract
1 teaspoon baking powder
1-1/3 cup gluten-free all-purpose baking flour mix

Directions

Preheat oven to 350° Fahrenheit . Mix wet ingredients (butter, honey, eggs and vanilla extract) together. Whisk dry ingredients together: sea salt, baking powder and flour. Slowly add dry mixture to wet until well-combined. Drop batter by rounded spoonfuls onto a greased baking sheet. Bake for 10-14 minutes or until edges are lightly browned.

Guacamole

Serves:	8
Prep time:	10 minutes
Special diets:	Body Ecology Diet, dairy-free, diabetic, egg-free, GAPS/SCD, gluten-free, Paleo, vegan, vegetarian
Meal type:	appetizers, sauces & dressings, snacks
Miscellaneous:	child-friendly, pre-preparable, serve cold
Occasion:	barbecue, casual party

Guacamole goes well with just about any savory dish – I use it on meats, beans, rice and veggies.

Ingredients

4 medium ripe avocados (peeled and pitted)
1 large red onion (small dice)
1 medium tomato (diced)
4 cloves garlic (minced)
1 bunch fresh cilantro (minced)
1 medium lime (juiced)
Sea salt (to taste)
1 medium jalapeno pepper (minced)

Directions

Mash avocados. Add in the onion, tomato, garlic, jalapeno, cilantro and lime juice; mix well. Add sea salt to taste.

Homemade Pediasure®

Serves:	4
Prep time:	5 minutes
Special diets:	dairy-free, diabetic, egg-free, gluten-free, vegan, vegetarian
Meal type:	drinks
Miscellaneous:	child-friendly, pre-preparable, serve cold

Ingredients

1 c. organic apple or pear juice
½ c. organic coconut milk
2 c. organic rice milk
4 scoops of Metagenics Ultracare for Kids (low-level vitamin supplement)
4 heaping tablespoons organic rice protein powder
2 tsp. organic vanilla powder
½ c. Udo's Oil (DHA & EPA)

Directions

Mix all ingredients except for oil in a blender. Blend oil in by hand. Thin out to desired consistency with organic rice milk.

Lamb with Figs and Oranges

Serves:	4
Prep time:	15 minutes
Cook time:	20 minutes
Total time:	35 minutes
Special diets:	dairy-free, egg-free, GAPS/SCD, gluten-free, Paleo
Meal type:	meats
Miscellaneous:	child-friendly, freezable, pre-preparable serve hot

I've created a simple yet flavorful dish of lamb with figs and oranges. It's Paleo-, GAPS- and SCD-legal.

Ingredients

1lb lamb (cut into 1-inch cubes)
1/2 teaspoon sea salt
1 tablespoon extra-virgin olive oil, coconut oil or ghee
4-5 cloves garlic (minced)
3 large oranges (juiced)
10 medium dried figs (chopped)
1/2 teaspoon Ceylon cinnamon

Directions

Marinate the lamb for a minimum of 2 hours in the juice of 2 oranges in the fridge. Toss the lamb with sea salt and brown in a large skillet over medium-high heat for a few minutes until all sides are brown. Remove from pan. Lower heat to medium low. Add olive oil and garlic to skillet and cook for 2-3 minutes. Add in the juice of the 3rd orange as well as the chopped figs. Cook until figs are softened, about 5 minutes. Return lamb to skillet. Add in cinnamon, stir, cook for another 2 minutes and serve.

Lentil Salad with Cilantro and Lime

Serves:	16
Prep time:	10 minutes
Cook time:	30 minutes
Total time:	40 minutes
Special diets:	dairy-free, diabetic, egg-free, GAPS/SCD, gluten-free, vegan, vegetarian
Meal type:	beans & legumes, side dishes
Miscellaneous:	pre-preparable

Cilantro, lime and red onion give a fresh twist to boring old lentils in this summer-salad recipe.

Ingredients

3 cups French lentils (soaked overnight, rinsed and drained)
5 cups filtered water or homemade stock
1 piece kombu (kelp)
1 bunch fresh flat-leaf parsley (minced)
1 bunch fresh cilantro (minced)
1 large red onion (diced)
1/2 cup extra-virgin olive oil
2 large limes (zested and juiced)
1 teaspoon sea salt

Directions

Bring lentils and kombu in broth to a boil; cover and simmer for 30 minutes or until tender. Drain and cool. Combine lentils with other ingredients in a large bowl.

Mashed Fauxtatoes

Serves:	4
Prep time:	5 minutes
Cook time:	15 minutes
Total time:	20 minutes
Special diets:	Body Ecology Diet, dairy-free, diabetic, egg-free, GAPS/SCD, gluten-free, Paleo, vegan, vegetarian
Meal type:	other vegetables, side dishes
Miscellaneous:	child-friendly, pre-preparable, serve hot

These GAPS, SCD and Paleo legal mashed fauxtatoes taste just like smooth and creamy mashed potatoes.

Ingredients

1 head cauliflower
1/4 cup ghee, butter or coconut oil (if you want a dairy-free version, use either ghee or coconut oil)
1/4 teaspoon sea salt
1/4 teaspoon garlic sea salt

Directions

Steam cauliflower until tender in steamer basket. In food processor or blender, blend all ingredients until smooth. Transfer to serving bowl. Serve immediately.

Navy Bean Chili

Serves:	4
Prep time:	5 minutes
Cook time:	2 hours, 15 minutes
Total time:	2 hours, 30 minutes
Special diets:	dairy-free, diabetic, egg-free, GAPS/SCD, gluten-free
Meal type:	beans & legumes, soups
Miscellaneous:	child-friendly, pre-preparable, serve hot

Ingredients

1 cup dried navy beans (soaked overnight, rinsed and drained)
3 cups filtered water or homemade broth
2 tablespoons ghee or extra-virgin olive oil
1 small kombu (kelp) piece
8oz pastured ground beef or bison
1 large onion (peeled and diced)
1 large red bell pepper (seeded and finely diced)
2 large carrots (peeled and diced)
2 stalks celery (diced)
3 large tomatoes (chopped)
3 cloves garlic (peeled and minced)
2 teaspoons ground cumin
1 teaspoon oregano
1 teaspoon chili powder
1 teaspoon sea salt
1/4 cup fresh flat-leaf parsley (minced)

Directions

Bring beans, water and kombu to boil. Skim off any foam. Lower heat, cover and simmer for 45 minutes or until tender. Add 1 tsp. sea salt; continue cooking for 1/2 hour. In a separate pan, melt ghee over medium heat. Saute' beef and onions. Add vegetables, garlic and spices; cook for 5-7 minutes. Combine sautéed vegetables and beef with the beans. Cover and cook another 10 minutes. Garnish with parsley.

Paleo Hummus

Serves:	4
Prep time:	5 minutes
Allergy:	tree nuts
Special diets:	dairy-free, diabetic, egg-free, GAPS/SCD, gluten-free, Paleo, vegan, vegetarian
Meal type:	appetizers, sauces & dressings, snacks
Miscellaneous:	child-friendly, pre-preparable, serve cold

Chickpeas and other legumes are not legal in the Paleo diet, but that doesn't mean you need to give up having hummus. Try this garlicky Paleo hummus as an appetizer, side dish or even as a dressing. I've substituted pine nuts and zucchini for chickpeas, so you get an extra serving of vegetables as a bonus!

Ingredients

1/4 cup pine nuts (soaked overnight and drained)
1/3 cup tahini
1 medium zucchini
1 large lemon (freshly squeezed)
1 clove garlic (minced)
1/4 teaspoon sea salt

Directions

Place all ingredients in a food processor or blender and blend until smooth.

Pecan Butter Kasha

Serves:	4
Prep time:	2 minutes
Cook time:	25 minutes
Total time:	27 minutes
Allergy:	tree nuts
Special diets:	dairy-free, diabetic, egg-free, gluten-free, vegan, vegetarian
Meal type:	breakfasts, grains
Miscellaneous:	child-friendly, freezable, pre-preparable, serve hot

Kasha is pre-roasted buckwheat, a gluten-free "grain" unrelated to wheat. This recipe is suitable for those following a gluten-free, dairy-free diet.

Ingredients

1 cup kasha (buckwheat groats)
1 tablespoon ghee, pastured butter or coconut oil
2 teaspoons maple syrup
3 dashes sea salt
4 tablespoons pecan butter

Directions

To cook kasha: Rinse and drain 1 cup of kasha 2-3 times. Add 2 cups of filtered water. Boil for 15 minutes. Remove from heat. Melt ghee, butter or coconut oil in a sauce pan. Add in the rest of the ingredients to kasha. Warm and stir thoroughly.

Sweet Green Smoothie

Serves:	4
Prep time:	5 minutes
Special diets:	dairy-free, diabetic, egg-free, gluten-free, GAPS/SCD, gluten-free, Paleo, vegan, vegetarian
Meal type:	juices & teas
Miscellaneous:	serve cold

Raw greens are an excellent source of true folate, which will help with methylation defects and thus, toxicity.

Ingredients

1/2 cup filtered water
1 medium cucumber
1 cup fresh dark-green lettuce
1/2 bunch parsley
1/2 bunch cilantro
3 ribs celery
1 cup strawberries or other berries

Directions

Place all ingredients into a blender. Blend until smooth.

Vegetable Broth

Serves:	16
Prep time:	5 minutes
Cook time:	24 hours
Total time:	24 hours, 5 minutes
Special diets:	Body Ecology Diet, dairy-free, diabetic, egg-free, GAPS/SCD, gluten-free, Paleo, vegan, vegetarian
Meal type:	soups
Miscellaneous:	child-friendly, freezable, pre-preparable, serve hot

Vegetables are sooo full of minerals. Where do you think the calcium in the milk that we're told to drink comes from?

Ingredients
6 large unpeeled carrots (cut into thirds)
2 large onions, unpeeled (roughly chopped)
1 large leek, white and green parts (roughly chopped)
1 bunch celery, including the heart (cut into thirds)
1 bunch kale (roughly chopped)
5 cloves garlic (smashed)
1/2 bunch fresh flat-leaf parsley
1 Strip kombu (kelp)
12 black peppercorns
4 whole allspice or juniper berries
2 bay leaves
8 quarts cold, filtered water
1 teaspoon sea salt

Directions
Rinse all of the vegetables well, including the kombu. In a crockpot, place all ingredients. Fill the pot with the water, set to low and let cook for 24 hours. Strain soup and discard vegetables. (I compost the leftover veggies.)

Wild Rice and Shiitake Stuffing

Serves:	12
Prep time:	15 minutes
Cook time:	1 hour
Total time:	1 hour, 15 minutes
Allergy:	tree nuts
Special diets:	dairy-free, diabetic, egg-free, gluten-free, vegan, vegetarian
Meal type:	grains, side dishes
Miscellaneous:	child-friendly, freezable, serve hot

Ingredients

3/4 cups wild rice (soaked overnight, rinsed and drained)
3/4 cups brown rice (soaked overnight, rinsed and drained)
1-1/2 cups cold, filtered water or homemade broth
1 piece kombu (kelp)
1 teaspoon sea salt
1 cup pecans (soaked, rinsed, drained, toasted and chopped)
3 tablespoons extra-virgin olive oil
1 medium onion (peeled and diced)
3 large celery ribs (diced)
8oz shiitake mushrooms (thinly sliced)
2 cloves garlic (peeled and minced)
1-1/2 tablespoon fresh sage or thyme (minced)
1 large carrot (peeled and diced)

Directions

Combine rice, broth, kombu and sea salt in a medium pot; boil over high heat. Cover, reduce heat to low and cook for 30 minutes. In a wide heavy skillet, heat 3 tablespoons oil over medium heat. Saute' onions for 5 minutes. Add carrots; saute' for 3 minutes. Stir in celery with a pinch of sea salt; cook for 5 minutes. Add garlic and sage; saute' another minute. Remove from pan. Wipe out pan; heat another 3 tablespoons oil over medium heat. Add in mushrooms; saute' until light brown. Add in other ingredients; combine.

RESOURCES

Articles

"Body Burden: The Pollution in Newborns", Environmental Working Group, www.ewg.org/research/body-burden-pollution-newborns

"The Dark Side of Wheat", Sayer Ji, www.greenmedinfo.com/page/dark-side-wheat-new-perspectives-celiac-disease-wheat-intolerance-sayer-ji

"Dirty Dozen Endocrine Disruptors", Environmental Working Group: www.ewg.org/research/dirty-dozen-list-endocrine-disruptors

"Hidden Sources of Gluten", www.webmd.com/diet/features/hidden-sources-of-gluten

"The Oiling of America", Mary Enig and Sally Fallon of the Weston A. Price Foundation,www.westonaprice.org/health-topics/the-oiling-of-america

"The Liver Files", Lynn Razaitis for the Weston A. Price Foundation, www.westonaprice.org/health-topics/the-liver-files

"The Ploy of Soy", Sally Fallon and Mary Enig of the Weston A. Price Foundation: www.westonaprice.org/health-topics/the-ploy-of-soy

"Vitamin Primer", the Weston A. Price Foundation http://www.westonaprice.org/vitamins-and-minerals/vitamin-primer

"Water Treatment Contaminants: Toxic Trash in Drinking Water", the Environmental Working Group

"What Causes Heart Disease?", Sally Fallon and Mary Enig of the Weston A. Price Foundation: www.westonaprice.org/modern-diseases/what-causes-heart-disease

"What Was in the World Trade Center Plume?", David Biello, *Scientific American*, Sep. 7, 2011

Books

Balcells, Cristy. *Living Well with Mitochondrial Disease: A Handbook for Patients, Parents, and Families.* Bethesda, MD: Woodbine House, Inc., 2012.

Beaman, Andrea. *The Whole Truth: Eating and Recipe Guide.* New York, NY: Andrea Beaman, 2006.

Billings, Kurt and Lee Ann. *Mold: The War Within.* Kodak, TN: Partners Publishing LLC, 2013.

Blaylock, Russell L., MD. *Excitoxins: The Taste That Kills.* Santa Fe, NM: Health Press, 1997.

Blaylock, Russell L., MD. *Health and Nutrition Secrets.* Albuquerque, NM: Health Press, 2006.

Blombert, Harald and Dempsey, Moira. *Movements that Heal.* Queensland, Australia: BookPal, 2011.

Bock, Kenneth, MD and Strauth, Cameron. *Healing the New Childhood Epidemics: Autism, ADHD, Asthma, and Allergies: The Groundbreaking Program for the 4-A Disorders.* New York, NY: Ballantine Books, 2008.

Bowthorpe, Janie A., M.Ed. *Stop the Thyroid Madness.* Florence, CO: Laughing Grape Publishing, 2008.

Breiner, Mark, DDS. *Whole-Body Dentistry: The Missing Piece to Better Health.* Quantum Health Press, LLC, 1999.

Brownstein, David, MD. *Iodine: Why You Need It, Why You Can't Live Without It.* West Bloomfield, MI: Medical Alternative Press, 2009.

Brownstein, David, MD. *Salt - Your Way to Health.* West Bloomfield, MI: Medical Alternative Press, 2006.

Campbell-McBride, Dr. Natasha. *Gut and Psychology Syndrome: Natural Treatment for Autism, Dyspraxia, A.D.D., Dyslexia, A.D.H.D., Depression Schizophrenia.* Amersham, England: Halstan & Co., Ltd., 2010.

Cave, Stephanie, MD. *What Your Doctor May Not Tell You About Your Children's Vaccinations.* New York, NY: Warner Books, Inc., 2001.

Christenson, Bryan. *The Fluoride Deception.* New York, NY: Seven Stories Press, 2004.

Cohen, Suzy, RPh. *Drug Muggers: Which Medications Are Robbing*

Your Body of Essential Nutrients--and Natural Ways to Restore Them. New York, NY: Rodale, 2011.

Colbin, Annemarie. *Food and Healing.* New York, NY: Ballantine Books, 1986.

Colburn, Theo, Dumanoski, Dianne and Meyers, John Peter. *Our Stolen Future: Are We Threatening Our Fertility, Intelligence, and Survival?--A Scientific Detective Story.* New York, NY: Plume, 1997.

Conroy, Helen and Hirsch, Laura. *Evolution of a Revolution: From Hope to Healing.* Rockport, MA: Team Thinking Moms' Revolution Press, 2014.

Conroy, Helen and Goes, Lisa Joyce. *The Thinking Moms' Revolution: Autism beyond the Spectrum: Inspiring True Stories from Parents Fighting to Rescue Their Children.* New York, NY: Skyhorse Publishing, 2013.

Coulter, Harris L. and Fisher, Barbara Loe. *A Shot in the Dark.* New York, NY: Plume, 1991.

Cowan, Stephen Scott, MD. *Fire Child, Water Child: How Understanding the Five Types of ADHD Can Help You Improve Your Child's Self-Esteem & Attention.* Oakland, CA: New Harbinger Publications, 2012.

Crook, William, MD. *The Yeast Connection: A Medical Breakthrough.* New York, NY: Vintage Books, 1986.

Cutler, Andrew Hall. *Amalgam Illness, Diagnosis and Treatment: What You Can Do to Get Better, What Your Doctor Can Do to Help.* Sammamish, WA: Andrew Hall Cutler, 1999.

Cutler, Ellen, DC and Tunkel, Richard, MD. *Clearing the Way to Health and Wellness: Reversing Chronic Conditions by Freeing the Body of Food, Environmental, and Other Sensitivities.* Bloomington, IN: iUniverse LLC, 2013.

D'Adamo, Peter. *Eat Right for Your Type: The Individualized Diet Solution to Staying Healthy, Living Longer & Achieving Your Ideal Weight.* New York, NY: G.P. Putnam's Sons, 1997.

Davis, William, MD. *Wheat Belly, Lose the Wheat, Lose the Weight, and Find Your Path Back to Health.* New York, NY: Rodale, 2011.

Dean, Carolyn, MD, ND. *The Magnesium Miracle.* New York, NY: Ballantine Books, 2007.

Dorfman, Kelly, MS, LND. *Cure Your Child with Food: The Hidden Connection Between Nutrition and Childhood Ailments.* New York, NY: Workman Publishing Co., Inc., 2013.

Erasmus, Udo. *Fats That Heal, Fats That Kill: The Complete Guide to Fats, Oils, Cholesterol and Human Health.* Burnaby, Canada: Alive Books, 1993.

Fallon, Sally and Enig, Mary. *Nourishing Traditions: The Cookbook that Challenges Politically Correct Nutrition and the Diet Dictocrats.* Washington, DC: NewTrends Publishing, Inc., 2001.

Farlow, Christine Hoza, DC. *Food Additives – A Shopper's Guide to What's Safe & What's Not.* KISS For Health Publishing, 2013.

Fife, Bruce, CN, ND. *The Coconut Oil Miracle.* New York, NY: Avery, 2004.

Fraser, Heather. *The Peanut Allergy Epidemic: What's Causing It and How to Stop It.* New York, NY: Skyhorse Publishing, 2011.

Gates, Donna. *The Body Ecology Diet: Recovering Your Health and Rebuilding Your Immunity.* Bogart, GA: B.E.D. Publications, 2007.

Gershon, Michael D., MD. *The Second Brain: A Groundbreaking New Understanding of Nervous Disorders of the Stomach and Intestine.* New York, NY: Harper Perennial, 1999.

Gittleman, Louise, PhD, CNS. *Guess What Came to Dinner?: Parasites and Your Health.* New York, NY: Avery Trade, 2001.

Gittleman, Ann Louise. *Zapped: Why Your Cell Phone Shouldn't Be Your Alarm Clock and 1,268 Ways to Outsmart the Hazards of Electronic Pollution.* New York, NY: HarperOne, 2011.

Goddard, Sally. *Reflexes, Learning and Behavior: A Window into the Child's Mind.* Eugene, OR: Fern Ridge Press, 2005.

Gotschall, Elaine. *Breaking the Vicious Cycle: Intestinal Health Through Diet.* Riccio, CA: The Kirkton Press, 1994.

Grandjean, Phillippe. *Only One Chance: How Environmental Pollution Impairs Brain Development -- and How to Protect the Brains of the Next Generation.* New York, NY: Oxford University Press, 2013.

Habakus, Louise Kuo, MA and Holland, Mary, JD, Editors. *Vaccine Epidemic: How Corporate Greed, Biased Science, and Coercive Government Threaten Our Human Rights, Our Health, and Our Children.* New York, NY: Skyhorse Publishing, 2012.

Halstead, Pauli. *Primal Cuisine: Cooking for the Paleo Diet.* Rochester, VT: Healing Arts Press, 2013.

Hamilton, Alissa. *Squeezed: What You Don't Know About Orange Juice.* New Haven, CT: Yale University Press, 2009.

Herbert, Martha, MD, PhD with Weintraub, Karen. *The Autism Revolution: Whole-Body Strategies for Making Life All It Can Be.* New York, NY: Ballantine Books, 2013.

Hirsch, Laura Lambert. *The Other Side of Autism.* Rainbow Books, 2012.

Hyman, Mark, MD. *The UltraMind Solution: Fix Your Broken Brain by Healing Your Body First.* New York, NY: Scribner, 2008.

Hyman, Mark, MD and Liponis, Mark, MD. *Ultraprevention.* New York, NY: Atria Books, 2005.

Irlen, Helen. *Reading by the Colors.* New York, NY: Perigree Trade, 2005.

Kaplan, Melvin. *Seeing Through New Eyes: Changing the Lives of Children with Autism, Asperger Syndrome and other Developmental Disabilities through Vision Therapy.* Philadelphia, PA: Jessica Kingsley Publishers, 2006.

Kennedy, Jr., Robert F., Editor. *Thimerosal: Let the Science Speak: The Evidence Supporting the Immediate Removal of Mercury – a Known Neurotoxin – from Vaccines.* New York, NY: Skyhorse Publishing, 2014.

Kharazzian, Datis, DHSc, DC, MS. *Why Do I Still Have Symptoms? when My Lab Tests Are Normal: a Revolutionary*

Breakthrough in Understanding Hashimoto's Disease and Hypothyroidism. Carlsbad, CA: Elephant Press LP, 2010.

Kranowitz, Carol Stock, MA. *The Out-of-Sync Child: Recognizing and Coping with Sensory Processing Disorder.* New York, NY: Perigree, 2005.

Lambert, Beth and Kobliner, Victoria, MS, RD. *A Compromised Generation: The Epidemic of Chronic Illness in America's Children.* Boulder, CO: Sentient Publications, 2010.

Langer, Stephen E., MD and Scheer, James F. *Solved: The Riddle of Illness.* New York, NY: McGraw-Hill, 2006.

Lemer, Patricia S., Ed. *Envisioning a Bright Future: Interventions That Work for Children and Adults with Autism Spectrum Disorder.* Santa Ana, CA: OEP Foundation, Inc., 2008.

Lemer, Patricia S. *Outsmarting Autism.* Tarentum, PA: Word Association Publishers, 2014.

Lennihan, Burke. *Your Natural Medicine Cabinet, A Practical Guide to Drug-Free Remedies for Common Ailments.* Cambridge, MA: GreenHealing Press, 2012.

Lipton, Bruce. *The Biology of Belief: Unleashing the Power of Consciousness, Matter, & Miracles.* Hay House, 2007.

Louv, Richard. *The Last Child in the Woods: Saving Our Children from Nature Deficit Disorder.* Chapel Hill, NC: Algonquin Books of Chapel Hill, 2008.

Margulis, Jennifer, PhD. *The Business of Baby: What Doctors Don't Tell You, What Corporations Try to Sell You, and How to Put Your Pregnancy, Childbirth, and Baby Before Their Bottom Line.* New York, NY: Scribner, 2013.

Matthews, Julie, CNC. *Nourishing Hope for Autism: Nutrition and Diet Guide for Healing Children: ADHD, Autism, Learning and Developmental Delays.* Healthful Living Media, 2008.

May, Jeffrey C. *My House Is Killing Me! The Home Guide for Families with Allergies and Asthma.* Baltimore, MD: The Johns Hopkins University Press, 2001.

Mercola, Joseph and Pearsall, Kendra Degen. *Sweet Deception: Why Splenda, NutraSweet, and the FDA May Be Hazardous to Your Health.* Nashville, TN: Thomas Nelson, Inc., 2006.

Miller, Lucy Jane, PhD, OTR. *Sensational Kids: Hope and Help for*

Children with Sensory Processing Disorder. New York, NY: Perigree, 2014.

Monastyrsky, Konstantin. *Fiber Menace: The Truth About the Leading Role of Fiber in Diet Failure, Constipation, Hemorrhoids, Irritable Bowel Syndrome, Ulcerative Colitis, Chron's Disease, and Colon Cancer.* Ageless Press, 2008.

Nakizawa, Donna Jackson. *The Autoimmune Epidemic.* New York, NY: Touchstone, 2008.

Nelson, Dr. Bradley. *The Emotion Code.* Mesquite, NV: Wellness Unmasked Publishing, 2007.

Ober, Clint, Sinatra, Stephen T., MD and Zucker, Martin. *Earthing: The Most Important Health Discovery Ever?* Laguna Beach, CA: Basic Health Publications, Inc., 2010.

O'Brien, Robyn. *The Unhealthy Truth: One Mother's Shocking Investigation into the Dangers of America's Food Supply– and What Every Family Can Do to Protect Itself.* New York, NY: Broadway Books, 2009.

Oden, Athena. *Ready Bodies, Learning Mind - A Key to Academic Success.* Spring Branch, TX: ReadyBodies, 2006

Olmsted, Dan and Blaxill, Mark. *The Age of Autism: Mercury, Medicine, and a Man-Made Epidemic.* New York, NY: Thomas Dunne Books, 2011.

Pacholok, Sally M., RN, BSN and Stuart, Jeffrey J., DO. *Could It Be B12? An Epidemic of Misdiagnoses.* Fresno, CA: Quill Driver Books, 2011.

Pangborn, Jon, PhD and Baker, Sidney M., MD. *Autism: Effective Biomedical Treatments.* Autism Research Institute, 2005.

Perlmutter, David, MD. *Grain Brain: The Surprising Truth about Wheat, Carbs, and Sugar – Your Brain's Silent Killers.* New York, NY: Little, Brown and Company, 2013.

Philpott, William K., MD and Kalita, Dwight K., PhD. *Brain Allergies: The Psychonutrient and Magnetic Connections.* Los Angeles, CA: Keats Publishing, 2000.

Pollan, Michael. *Food Rules: An Eater's Manual.* New York, NY: Penguin Books, 2009.

Pollan, Michael. *The Omnivore's Dilemma.* New York, NY: Penguin Books, 2009.

Prasad, Raman. *Recipes for the Specific Carbohydrate Diet.* Beverly, MA: Fair Winds Press, 2008.

Price, Weston A. and the Price-Pottenger Nutrition Foundation, *Nutrition and Physical Degeneration.* Washington, DC: Price Pottenger Nutrition, 2009.

Rapp, Doris, MD. *Is This Your Child?.* New York, NY: William Morrow Paperbacks, 1992.

Rogers, Sherry, MD. *The Cholesterol Hoax.* Sarasota, FL: Prestige Publishing, 2008.

Rogers, Sherry, MD. *Detoxify or Die.* Sarasota, FL: Sand Key Company, Inc., 2002.

Rogers, Sherry, MD. *How to Cure Diabetes.* Sarasota, FL: Prestige Publishing, 2012.

Rogers, Sherry, MD. *Pain Free in 6 Weeks.* Sarasota, FL: Prestige Publishing, 2001.

Ross, Julia, MA. *The Diet Cure: The 8-Step Program to Rebalance Your Body Chemistry and End Food Cravings, Weight Gain, and Mood Swings – Naturally.* New York, NY: Penguin Books, 2012.

Ross, Julia, MA. *The Mood Cure: The 4-Step Program to Take Control of Your Emotions – Today.* New York, NY: Penguin Books, 2002.

Salatin, Joel. *Folks, This Ain't Normal: A Farmer's Advice for Happier Hens, Healthier People and a Better World.* New York, NY: Center Street, 2012.

Sears, Robert W., MD, FAAP. The *Autism Book: What Every Parent Needs to Know About Early Detection, Treatment, Recovery, and Prevention (Sears Parenting Library).* New York, NY: Little, Brown and Company, 2010.

Sears, Robert W., MD, FAAP. *The Vaccine Book: Making the Right Decision for Your Child (Sears Parenting Library).* New York, NY: Little, Brown and Company, 2011.

Sircus, Mark, DC. *Sodium Bicarbonate – Full Medical Review.* International Medical Veritas Association, 2010.

Smith, Jeffrey M. *Genetic Roulette: The Documented Health Risks of Genetically Modified Foods*. Fairfield, IA: Yes! Books, 2007.

Smith, Jeffrey. *Seeds of Deception: Exposing Industry and Government Lies About the Safety of the Genetically Engineered Foods You're Eating*. Fairfield, IA: Yes! Books, 2003.

Smith, Rick and Lourie, Bruce. *Slow Death by Rubber Duck: The Secret Danger of Everyday Things*. Berkeley, CA: Counterpoint, 2009.

Smits, Tinus, MD. *Autism, Beyond Despair: CEASE Therapy, Homeopathy Has the Answers*. Emryss Publishers, 2010.

Tam, Michelle and Fong, Henry. *Nom Nom Paleo: Food for Humans*. Kansas City, MO: Andrews McMeel Publishing, 2013.

Thompson, Robert, MD and Barnes, Kathleen. *The Calcium Lie: What Your Doctor Doesn't Know Could Kill You*. InTruth Press, 2008.

Walker, Danielle. *Against All Grain: Delectable Paleo Recipes to Eat Well and Feel Great*. Victory Belt Publishing, 2013.

Warshowsky, Joel H. *How Behavioral Optometry Can Unlock Your Child's Potential: Identifying and Overcoming Blocks to Concentration, Self-Esteem and School Success with Vision Therapy*. Philadelphia, PA: Jessica Kingsley Publishers, 2012.

Wilson, Dr. James O. and Wright, Dr. Jonathan. *Adrenal Fatigue: The 21st Century Syndrome*. Petaluma, CA: Smart Publications, 2001.

Winston, David and Steven Maimes. *Adaptogens: Herbs for Strength, Stamina and Stress Relief*. Rochester, VT: Healing Arts Press, 2007.

Weissbluth, Marc, MD. *Healthy Sleep Habits, Happy Child*. New York, NY: Random House Publishing, Inc., 2003.

Wahls, Terry, MD. *Minding Your Mitochondria*. Iowa City, IA: TZ Press, LLC, 2010.

Wolf, Robb. *The Paleo Solution: The Original Human Diet*. Victory Belt Publishing, 2010.

DVDs/Films/Videos

Angelfish Therapy (aquatic occupational therapy) DVD training products: www.angelfishtherapy.com
Bought
Canary Kids Project: www.canarykidsmovie.com
Farmageddon
Food Matters
Genetic Roulette
GMO OMG
The Greater Good
King Corn
Masgutova Method books and DVDs for reflex integration: www.masgutova.com
Move, Play, Thrive for neurodevelopmental movement: www.moveplaythrive.com
Semper Fi: Always Faithful
The Thyroid-Autism Connection, Dr. Raphael Kellman at the 2012 AutismOne Conference: www.autismone.org content/thyroid-autism-connection-2
Trace Amounts
Under Our Skin

Newsletters

Above the Fold, Environmental Health News: www.environmentalhealthnews.org
Body Ecology newsletter: www.bodyecology.com
International Medical Veritas Association: www.drsircus.com
Mercola: www.mercola.com
Rodale Daily News: www.rodalenews.com
Total Wellness Newsletter, Sherry Rogers, MD: www.prestigepublishing.com

Websites

Agency for Toxic Substances & Disease Registry: www.atsdr.cdc.gov
Andrew Weil, MD: www.drweil.com

Angelfish Therapy: www.angelfishtherapy.com
Annemarie Colbin: www.foodandhealing.com
Auditory Integration Training Services: www.aithelps.com
Autism Action Network: www.autismactionnetwork.org
Autism File Magazine: www.autismfile.com
BioSET: www.bioset.net
Body Ecology: www.bodyecology.com
Breaking the Vicious Cycle: breakingtheviciouscycle.info
Campaign for Real Milk: www.realmilk.com
Canary Kids Project: www.canarykidsmovie.com
CEASE Therapy: www.cease-therapy.com
Cheeseslave: www.cheeseslave.com
College of Optometrists in Vision Development:
www.covd.org
Cornucopia Institute: www.cornucopia.org
CureMito: www.curemito.org
Detoxinista: www.detoxinista.com
Developmental Delay Resources: www.devdelay.org
Dirty Electricity: www.dirtyelectricity.com
Doctor's Data: www.doctorsdata.com
Dr. David Clark's Brain Based Blog: www.drclark.typepad.com
Dr. Ellen Cutler: www.drellencutler.com
Earthing: www.earthing.com
Electric Sense: www.electricsense.com
Empowered Sustenance: www.empoweredsustenance.com
Environmental Working Group: www.ewg.org
Epidemic Answers: www.epidemicanswers.org
EWG Cleaners Database: www.ewg.org/guides/cleaners
Family Hope Center: www.familyhope.org
Feingold Diet Program for ADHD: www.feingold.org
Fluoride Action Network: www.fluoridealert.org
FODMAP Friendly Food Program: www.fodmaps.com
FoodBabe: www.foodbabe.com
Food Renegade: www.foodrenegade.com
Genova Diagnostics: www.gdx.net
Greater Good Movie: www.greatergoodmovie.org
Great Plains Laboratory: www.greatplainslaboratory.com

GreenMedInfo: www.greenmedinfo.com
GreenToys: www.greentoys.com
Gut Sense: www.gutsense.org
Gutsy: www.mygutsy.com
Healers Who Share: www.healerswhoshare.com
Healthy Child, Healthy World: www.healthychild.org
HealthyStuff.org: www.healthystuff.org
The Honest Company: www.honest.com
Igenex: www.igenex.com
Immunitrition: www.immunitrition.com
Institute for Functional Medicine:
www.functionalmedicine.org
Institute for Integrative Nutrition:
www.integrativenutrition.com
Institute for Responsible Technology:
www.responsibletechnology.org
International Medical Veritas Association: www.drsircus.com
John Douillard's LifeSpa: www.lifespa.com
Joseph Mercola: www.mercola.com
Julie Matthews Nourishing Hope: www.nourishinghope.com
Klinghardt Academy: www.klinghardtacademy.com
Lawrence A. Kotlow, DDS, PC: www.kidsteeth.com
LL'S Magnetic Clay: www.magneticclay.com
Loving Our Guts: www.lovingourguts.com/tongue-tie-2/
Mark's Daily Apple: www.marksdailyapple.com
Mark Hyman, MD: www.drhyman.com
Maria Rickert Hong: www.mariarickerthong.com
Masgutova Method: www.masgutova.com
Mito Action: www.mitoaction.org
Mommypotamus: www.mommypotamus.com
Mount Sinai Children's Environmental Health Center:
www.mountsinai.org/patient-care/service-areas/children/areas-of-care/childrens-environmental-health-center
Move, Play, Thrive for neurodevelopmental movement and reflex integration: www.moveplaythrive.com
MTHFR.net: www.mthfr.net

Nambudripad's Allergy Elimination Techniques:
www.naet.com
Natural Gourmet Institute: www.naturalgourmetinstitute.com
National Vaccine Information Center: www.nvic.org
No Amalgam: www.noamalgam.com
Organic Consumers Association: www.organicconsumers.org
PubMed: www.pubmed.org
Questioning Answers:
www.questioning-answers.blogspot.com
Raphael Kellman, MD: www.raphaelkellmanmd.com
Ready Bodies, Learning Minds: www.readybodies.com
Richard Louv: www.richardlouv.com
Robyn O'Brien: www.robynobrien.com
Rodale News: www.rodalenews.com
SCD Lifestyle: www. scdlifestyle.com
Science Daily: www.sciencedaily.com
Shopper's Guide to Pesticides in Produce, Environmental
Working Group: www.ewg.org/foodnews/
Skin Deep Cosmetics Database: www.ewg.org/skindeep
SPD Foundation: www.spdfoundation.net
SurvivingMold.com: www.survivingmold.com
Talk About Curing Autism: www.tacanow.org
The Thinking Moms' Revolution:
www.thinkingmomsrevolution.com
Tongue Tie: www.tonguetie.net.
Unblind My Mind: www.unblindmymind.com
United Mitochondrial Disease Foundation: www.umdf.org
VaxTruth: www.vaxtruth.org
Weston A. Price Foundation: www.westonaprice.org
The Yasko Protocol by Dr. Amy Yasko. www.dramyyasko.com
Yeast Connection: www.yeastconnection.com

INDEX

B

C

D

E

F

G

H

I

J

N

O

P

Q

R

S

T

U

V

W

X

Y

Z

ABOUT THE AUTHOR

I am a former Wall Street research analyst who is now a Certified Holistic Health Counselor who specializes in recovery from symptoms of autoimmune, neurological and digestive disorders, and I have recovered my sons from Sensory Processing Disorder, asthma and acid reflux.

I am a Board Member, Media Director and Blogger for Epidemic Answers (www.epidemicanswers.org), a 501(c)3 non-profit whose goal is to let parents know recovery is possible from autism, ADHD, SPD, allergies, asthma, autoimmune, Lyme and more.

I am also the Media Director for Epidemic Answers' Canary Kids Project (www.canarykidsmovie.com), which will be documenting the potential recovery of 14 children with autism, ADHD, asthma, atopic dermatitis, juvenile rheumatoid arthritis, mood disorders and type 2 diabetes as they receive free biomedical doctor visits, treatments, supplements, therapies, foods and lab tests for 18 months.

Website:	www.MariaRickertHong.com
Facebook:	Maria Rickert Hong Nutritional Healing
Twitter:	@mariarickert
Google+:	+Mariarickerthong
LinkedIn:	Maria Rickert Hong, CHHC, AADP
List.ly:	list.ly/maria.rickert.hong
Pinterest:	www.pinterest.com/mariarickert
Slideshare:	www.slideshare.net/mrickert
YouTube:	Maria Rickert Hong

Almost Autism:

Facebook:	www.facebook.com/almostautism
Twitter:	@almostautism

CPSIA information can be obtained at www.ICGtesting.com
Printed in the USA
LVOW10s0855041015

456839LV00021B/1084/P